THE MOUNTAIN ROSE HERBS

Book of Natural Body Care

THE MOUNTAIN ROSE HERBS

Book of Natural Body Care

68 Simple Recipes for Health and Beauty

Timber Press
Portland, Oregon

Published in 2024 by Timber Press, Inc., a subsidiary of Workman Publishing Co., Inc.,
a subsidiary of Hachette Book Group, Inc.
1290 Avenue of the Americas
New York, New York 10104

timberpress.com

Printed in China on responsibly sourced paper
Text and cover design by Emily Dubin
The publisher is not responsible for websites (or their content) that are not owned by the publisher.
The Hachette Speakers Bureau provides a wide range of authors for speaking events. To find
out more, go to hachettespeakersbureau.com or email HachetteSpeakers@hbgusa.com.

ISBN 978-1-64326-335-9
Catalog records for this book are available from the Library of Congress
and the British Library.

All photos by Mountain Rose Herbs

Contents

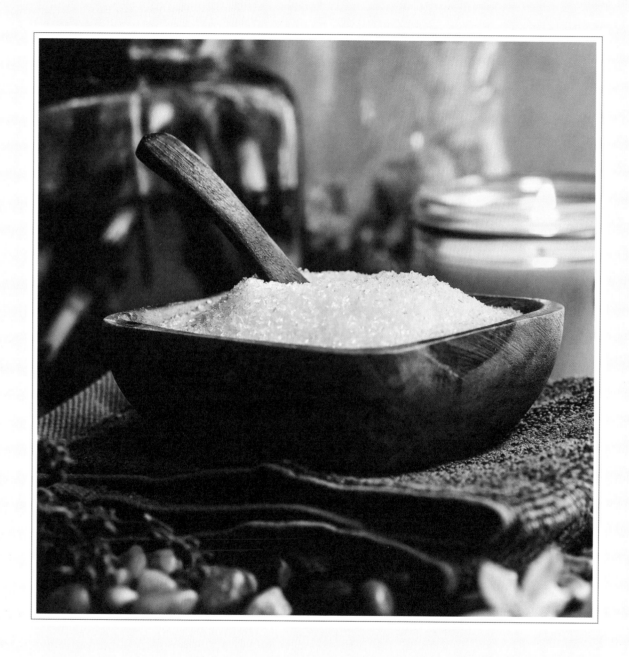

Preface

People, plants, and planet are more important than profit. This seemingly simple principle is the bedrock on which Mountain Rose Herbs is built, the foundational philosophy that has guided us for more than thirty-five years. From the beginning, we have been committed to the fundamental belief that it is our honor and our responsibility to live and work by ethical principles in ways that caretake our planet. We understand that at the end of the day, sustainable quality of life for all of us hinges on how we tend to our watersheds; how we nurture our soils, water, and air; how we grow and distribute the food we eat and the herbs we love. This is why we advocate relentlessly for sustainable organic agriculture, native plants, and fair trade.

Mountain Rose Herbs was founded in 1987 by Rosemary Gladstar, the "godmother of herbalism." The company began as a small mail-order business in northern California that provided supplies for students at the California School of Herbal Studies. When Rosemary moved on to Vermont to cofound Sage Mountain Botanical Sanctuary, other herbalists took up the reins of Mountain Rose Herbs. For many years, we worked out of a home and two-car garage, developing and formulating our first line of natural products, including teas, face creams, aroma sprays, and oils. By the 1990s, our reputation as a premier source for the finest ethically harvested botanicals and organic formulations was growing among herbalists and natural foods stores.

In 2000, under the direction of owner and environmental activist Shawn Donnille, we obtained official organic certification, built the first Mountain Rose Herbs retail website, and officially outgrew our California facilities. In 2001, we made an epic move to Oregon to be closer to our farm operators, wild harvesters, and processors. This move allowed us to create a first-of-its-kind full-time laboratory and quality-control department. We became a certified processor through Oregon Tilth in 2002.

From these humble beginnings, Mountain Rose Herbs has grown into one of the largest distributors of organic dried herbs, DIY ingredients, essential oils, teas, and spices in North America.

As we have grown, we have also expanded the work we do with people, plants, and planet in mind. We were the first Oregon company to receive TRUE Zero Waste Facility certification; the TRUE program is a whole-system approach aimed at changing how materials flow through society and encourages the redesign of resource life cycles so that all products are reused. We also invest deeply in the Mountain Rose River Project to help restore local riparian ecosystems. And we care for our employees' health—and that of the planet too—by providing an Alternative Commute Bonus for all our employees who walk, bike, bus, or carpool to work. These and other small acts of change add up to measurable benefits for all.

Sharing our three-plus decades of expertise and our unflinching commitment to sourcing the finest botanicals in the most ethical and respectful manner is at the heart of this book. As you peruse these body and skincare recipes, please know that they are rooted in the ancient traditions that humans have turned to for millennia: in the profoundly healing beauty of nature and the natural gifts of the botanical world.

Introduction

As with any craft, it's important to begin experimenting with DIY body care recipes only after you have learned the foundational knowledge that will help ensure your safety and success. In the first sections of this book, you'll find the fundamental information, concepts, and skills that every recipe in this book is built upon. Spending time here will give you the tools and flexibility to make these recipes your own.

The recipes in this book were chosen with the beginning body care crafter in mind. For instance, all of these recipes use dried herbs unless otherwise stated, because—unlike fresh plant material—dried herbs do not introduce water, which can significantly reduce shelf life. Additionally, the recipes included here use natural antioxidants when necessary to add stability to homemade skin and body care products, and some formulations will require refrigeration. The key to maximizing shelf life is understanding your ingredients and process.

One of the main reasons to create natural and organic body care products is to avoid the synthetic chemicals found in commercial options that allow products to sit on shelves for months or even years. With this in mind, understand that while we can add some preservation properties to our creations, we cannot expect our handcrafted shampoos, rinses, and creams to have the same shelf life as mass-produced, commercial products. Our advice is to craft in small batches and share with friends and family. Use it up while the ingredients are fresh!

Preservation is a topic that's vast enough to fill its own book. If you enjoy these recipes and are interested in learning more about crafting body care products that require more stabilization for a longer shelf life, we recommend taking advanced certified courses on formulating natural body care recipes so that you can create safe products to use and share.

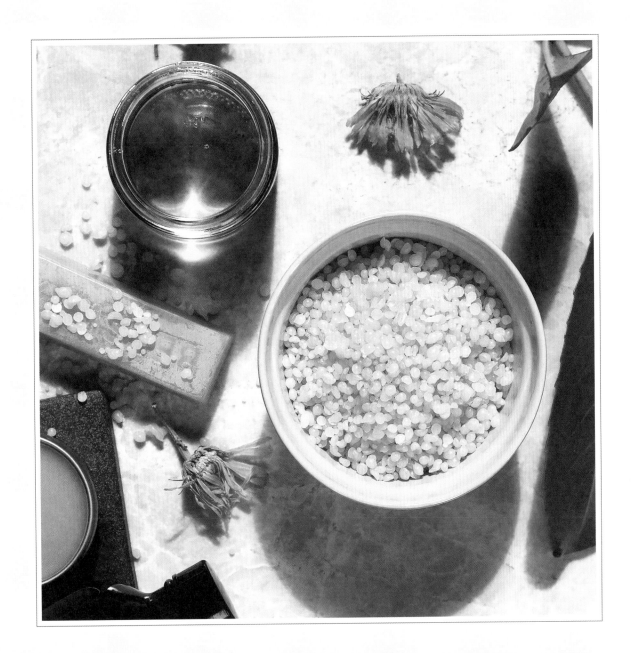

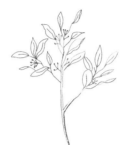

Foundational Knowledge

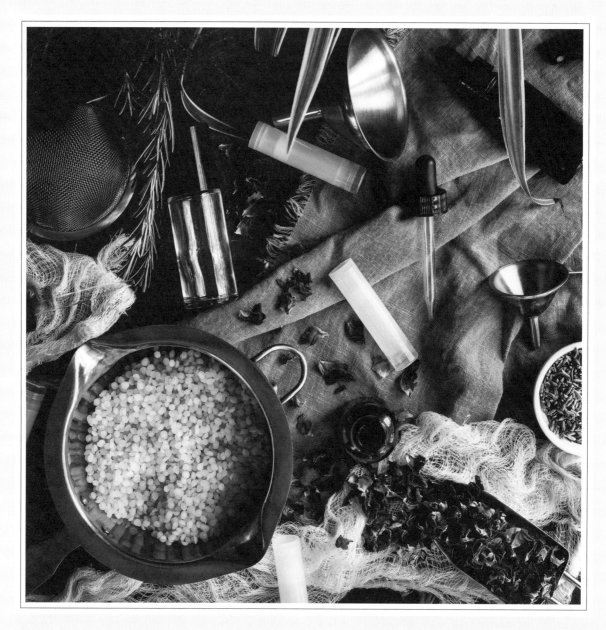

*Keeping a basic set of tools and containers on hand
allows you to craft whenever you're inspired.*

Tools & Supplies

Having the right tools sets you up for success when making body care products. Luckily, many of these tools are easy to find and are not costly. It is a good practice to keep your body care formulating supplies separate from your cooking implements since some of the pots and pans may develop hard-to-clean spots from ingredients like beeswax or propolis. For a truly sustainable setup, check your local second-hand store; many of these tools can be found used.

Choosing Tool Materials

Stainless steel Many herbalists prefer using stainless steel because it is practical, easy to work with, easy to clean, and sturdy enough for years of use. It is our number 1 go-to.

Glass Another material that many sustainability-minded crafters reach for is glass. Like stainless steel, glass is easy to clean and can stand the test of time. One of the downsides to glass is that it often breaks when dropped, and dropping is more likely when working with oils, butters, and other slippery materials.

Wood Some of us choose to work with wood utensils because of the natural and earthy feel and sustainable options. However, wood is not easy to clean because it is porous and is also prone to damage if left in liquids.

Plastic Although plastic is our least favorite material to work with, many herbalists appreciate that it is readily available and it is often inexpensive. However, it's not ideal when working with hot liquids and, because plastic is porous, it is difficult to thoroughly clean.

Building a DIY Toolkit

Spare pot and pans devoted to DIY crafts Many recipes include ingredients that may be difficult to clean, so it's a good idea to use a spare pot that you are not attached to.

Designated set of various sized bowls These are handy for premeasuring ingredients and for having on hand when you need to mix different volumes of materials.

Double boiler For the same reason that spare pots are a good idea, a double boiler designated for craft use is also a good idea. It will ensure that ingredients melt more evenly and do not burn, which can happen when placed on the direct heat of the burner.

Small stainless steel funnels Small funnels are helpful when filling smaller vessels with ingredients or finished products. We prefer using stainless steel because it is easy to clean.

Cotton tea net or cotton muslin bags With their small mesh size, these are incredibly helpful for filtering ingredients. They can even help to strain powders.

Hand mixer   Although most recipes can be mixed by hand, an electric hand mixer may make things a bit easier, especially when blending creams and butters.

Measuring spoons and cups   You may already own kitchen measuring spoons and cups, but it's a good idea to make sure you are working with a full set. You should have ⅛ teaspoon through 1 Tablespoon, and you'll want measuring vessels with partial cup measurements for both dry and liquid ingredients.

Set of kitchen implements   Having a designated spoon, fork, and knife will come in handy for those moments when you need another quick stir, poke, or cut. These can be easily procured at a second-hand store, so you won't have to worry about ruining utensils you care about.

Chopsticks   While not a common thing that most people keep in their toolkit, our team has found these very helpful for stirring, pouring, and scraping that may be needed along the way.

Rubber spatula   If you don't want to waste any of your finished product, a rubber spatula is a crucial implement to have on hand.

Bottles, jars, tins, and tubes   You will also need a place to store your formulations. Choosing quality containers that can be reused is helpful to keep long-term costs down. Be sure to thoroughly wash, sanitize, and dry your vessels before use. Some of the handiest receptacles are:

› Bottles with dropper tops
› Bottles with screw caps
› Bottles with treatment pumps
› Glass jars
› Lip balm tubes
› Roll-top glass bottles
› Air-tight storage jars

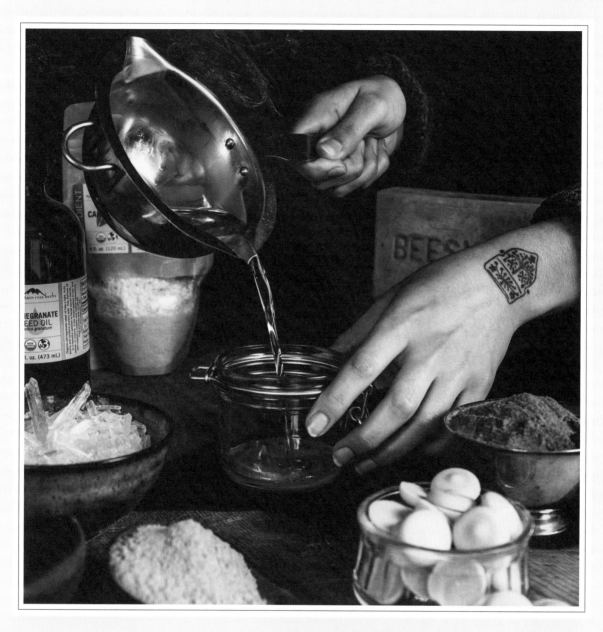

A good starting point is to learn about some of the most popular foundational herbs and essential oils for skin and hair care.

Guide to DIY Ingredients

One of the reasons many of us try to get away from conventional body care products is to avoid the synthetic ingredients they contain. Some of these ingredients, as well as the additives that are used to increase shelf life, have been known to cause allergic reactions and health problems and are often toxic to plant and animal life when they leach into the soil or water. Additionally, commercial skin and hair care products are often packaged in plastic containers that cannot be recycled or reused. Every year, people purchase millions of products in plastic bottles that end up in landfills or incinerators or find their way into our waterways, oceans, and wild areas, where they degrade and release toxins for hundreds of years. For those of us who value the natural world, going DIY can be an all-around win for our bodies, our health, and our planet.

As you purchase ingredients to make and customize your DIY body care recipes, remember that whatever you put on your skin is going to be absorbed into your body. Using high-quality and pure ingredients is how you ensure that what you create is effective and safe for use.

We believe that organic agriculture and sustainable sourcing are key to quality and purity. These practices are also fundamental in protecting ecosystems. All plants absorb nutrients and water through root uptake, a process known as bioaccumulation. Conventional farms use synthetic agricultural fertilizers, pesticides, and herbicides. These chemicals are absorbed by the crops they produce, and there is no way to wash them away. When you use conventionally grown herbs that are farmed in this manner, you are putting those chemicals on and in your body. Synthetic chemicals and fertilizers also destroy billions of life forms found in the soil and strip the land of the essential building blocks of life. Committing to organic botanicals that are sustainably grown, harvested, and processed helps protect you, your loved ones, and the planet we call home.

Know Your Ingredients

Purchase ingredients that are certified organic and/or sourced from a supplier you trust. This practice helps you avoid pesticides and other toxins that plants can take up and that can then be concentrated in oils and formulations. Keep in mind that some wild harvested plants, as well as plants cultivated without chemicals, may lack organic certification but may still be an excellent choice.

Purchase small amounts to start. We believe botanicals are precious and, in many cases—especially with essential oils—a small amount can go a long way. Plus, some herbs and oils can be pricey, so starting small and discovering what you love makes sense before purchasing large amounts.

Memorize a little Latin to ensure you are getting exactly what you want. A plant may be sold under the same common name, even though it is actually from a different genus and species: for example, both *Berberis aquifolium* and *Curcuma longa* are called golden root, but these plants aren't used in the same way. Learning the common name and the Latin name helps you know you've gotten the correct plant.

Learn the differences among plant parts. A plant's leaf or root or bark or essential oil may bring very different properties and aromas to your creation, so it is important to know and purchase the part you want.

Consider extraction methods and refinement techniques. If purchasing an oil or butter, was it made by cold pressing (no heat), expeller pressing (minimal heat), or solvent extraction? Is it unrefined, physically refined (no solvents used), or chemically refined?

Herbs and Essential Oils for Hair and Skin Care

For thousands of years, people have harnessed the power of pure, natural botanicals to support healthy hair and skin. The herbs and oils we highlight here are just a few that have proven themselves over time to be some of our best allies. You can use fresh or dried herbs to make luscious, handcrafted topical formulations customized for your particular goals. Using the essential oils of your favorite herbs is an excellent option as well and can give you a more shelf-stable and aromatic end product.

FAVORITE HERBS FOR HAIR AND SKIN CARE

Calendula (*Calendula officinalis*) This plant's flowers are renowned for their gentle, skin-nourishing properties. They are an excellent addition to general skin and scalp conditioning formulations and bring soothing, hydrating attributes to protective salves, diaper balms, and skin care recipes designed to neutralize occasional irritations, itchiness, and dryness.

Chamomile (*Matricaria chamomilla*) Used by ancient civilizations for thousands of years, this gentle flower is a perfect addition to body and hair care formulations, particularly in those designed to soothe minor irritation and redness. Chamomile is an excellent choice for cleansing washes and serums.

Chickweed (*Stellaria media*) Considered energetically cooling and moistening, chickweed is an excellent source of minerals that are ideal for skin washes and soothing, hydrating formulations that encourage a soft, smooth appearance. Chickweed is particularly ideal for relieving general skin discomfort.

Horsetail (*Equisetum arvense*) Because of its silica content, horsetail helps deliver nutrients to hair follicles and the scalp. It is also known to stimulate scalp circulation, providing extra blood for healthy follicles and strong hair. These qualities make horsetail a good choice for all hair types, although it is particularly helpful when the scalp and hair are oily. Horsetail's silica and collagen content makes it beneficial for the skin as well. An excellent choice for all skin types, it is especially cleansing and soothing for skin issues caused by occasional inflammation. The mineral content in horsetail is also beneficial in strengthening weak nails.

Lavender (*Lavandula angustifolia* or *Lavandula ×intermedia*) These plants have been some of the most beloved herbs for hair and skin care for thousands of years. In shampoos and rinses, lavender stimulates circulation, which supports a healthy scalp and strong hair for all hair types. It is also effective at soothing occasional scalp conditions like irritation and dandruff. Lavender is also often found in soaps, salves, soaks, and other skin care formulations because it supports and refreshes skin while providing a calming floral scent. It is an excellent choice for all skin types and is particularly good for cleaning pores and soothing isolated irritation and inflammation.

Marshmallow root (*Althaea officinalis*) The mucilaginous quality of marshmallow root coats, moisturizes, and softens hair, making it a wonderful addition in conditioners, detanglers, and serums for all hair types. It is particularly beneficial for dry and/or brittle hair. Formulations with marshmallow root are also helpful if you experience unruly, fly-away hair.

Nettle leaf (*Urtica dioica*) The leaves of nettle are astringent and contain silica and minerals, making them beneficial to both hair and skin. An excellent choice in cleansing washes and facial toners for all skin types, the plant's astringent properties make it an especially good choice for dry skin, reducing redness, balancing the production of sebum (the oil that our skin naturally produces), and supporting healthy skin elasticity. Nettle is also particularly useful in hair care formulations that stimulate circulation at the scalp and support hair follicle health. It is an excellent choice for overall hair health and soothing occasional scalp irritation. Nettle is wonderful for all hair types and can help keep sebum in balance, so hair doesn't become too dry or oily.

Peppermint (*Mentha ×piperita*) Menthol and menthone are the two primary compounds in peppermint. They provide a refreshing, revitalizing quality when added to hair and skin care formulations. Good for all skin types, peppermint's natural cleansing, cooling qualities are particularly good for oily skin and soothing for occasional skin irritation. In hair care products, peppermint can stimulate the scalp and increase circulation to give an invigorating boost to healthy hair follicles and is also an excellent choice to address issues involving dandruff or an itchy scalp.

Rosemary (*Rosmarinus officinalis*) Long used to maintain overall hair and skin health, rosemary is an excellent choice for all hair and skin types. It is often used in skin care recipes intended to balance sebum and soothe occasional irritation and redness. Rosemary is also known to stimulate circulation at the scalp, which in turn supports hair growth and shine and can help to reduce dandruff and ease scalp conditions.

FAVORITE ESSENTIAL OILS FOR HAIR AND SKIN CARE

Carrot seed (*Daucus carota*) A favorite in skin and scalp care recipes, carrot seed essential oil is appropriate for all skin and hair types and provides important vitamins, including collagen-supporting vitamin C.

Its vitamin E content is moisturizing, which makes it especially popular in recipes for sensitive or mature skin, as well as recipes addressing occasional dryness and irritations.

Frankincense (*Boswellia carteri*) With its lush and enticing aromatics, frankincense is beloved in perfumery. In hair care products, this essential oil stimulates circulation to the scalp and hair follicles, which supports healthy hair growth. Frankincense is also popular around the world in cosmetic formulations for all skin types, where it is used to help smooth and tone skin and to clear occasional blemishes.

Helichrysum (*Helichrysum italicum*) Excellent for all skin and hair types, helichrysum essential oil brings an earthy, sweet, floral aroma to a wide variety of formulations. This cleansing, popular oil is noted for supporting collagen and elastin, which helps to smooth blemishes and provide a healthy complexion. This essential oil also excels at soothing skin discomfort and itchiness for sensitive or irritated scalps.

Lavender (*Lavandula angustifolia*) Not only does the unmistakable sweet, floral, and herbal aroma of lavender essential oil appeal to most people, it is also helpful in maintaining healthy skin and scalp. This oil is excellent for all skin types and is found in body care and perfume formulations around the world. Because

it is non-comedogenic, it is particularly supportive of oily skin issues. Additionally, this oil is used to assist with occasional dandruff or scalp dryness.

Neroli (*Citrus aurantium*) With its beautifully delicate and sweet floral aroma, neroli essential oil is popular in perfume blends and skin and hair care products. It is a good choice for all skin types. Neroli is both hydrating and deeply moisturizing, with natural sebum-balancing qualities that make it an excellent choice in skin and scalp care recipes intended to address dry, sensitive, or mature skin.

Peppermint (*Mentha ×piperita*) The natural cleansing and refreshing qualities of peppermint essential oil help to balance excessive oils, which makes it ideal in formulations for normal to oily skin and hair. Its invigorating qualities also improve circulation in the scalp, which in turn enlivens and invigorates hair follicles and can help ease scalp itchiness.

Rosemary (*Rosmarinus officinalis*) This essential oil is deeply hydrating and can be used for all hair and skin types. Rosemary is often included in products intended to reduce skin blemishes, irritation, and redness, and it is also excellent in recipes that address occasional scalp irritation and itchiness. Rosemary essential oil is noted for its ability to support a healthy scalp and, in turn, hair growth.

Tea tree (*Melaleuca alternifolia*) This essential oil is known for its fresh, camphoraceous scent. Although tea tree essential oil is good for all skin types, it is especially soothing for sensitive or irritated scalps, as well as skin discomfort and itchiness. It is used to deeply cleanse and carry away impurities, dirt, and the accumulation of residues, so is often found in products that address oily skin and blemishes and in dandruff shampoos and hair care products intended to create lift and bounce.

Virginia cedarwood (*Juniperus virginiana*) This essential oil is good for most hair and skin types. Like lavender, Virginia cedarwood essential oil is helpful in maintaining overall skin and scalp health, but imparts an earthy, more grounded aroma. It has been reported to assist with balanced oil production.

Ylang ylang (*Cananga odorata*) The intoxicating aroma of ylang ylang essential oil makes it a favorite in perfumery as well as skin and hair care recipes. It is often used for stimulating hair growth and is touted as being a great stimulant for sebum and oil production, making it helpful for dry skin conditions and in managing dry, brittle hair and preventing breakage and further thinning.

Essential Oil Storage and Safety

Plants create resins and volatile aromatic oils to attract pollinators, warn predators, and to protect themselves against disease. The product called essential oil is this aromatic substance that is gathered and concentrated through methods like steam distillation, water distillation, and cold press extraction.

Essential oils can bring remarkable herbal support to skin and hair care formulations. However, it is important to use these highly concentrated aromatics safely because they enter our bloodstream and brain through our olfactory system and skin. While this ability allows the plant properties to create positive changes within our bodies, it also means essential oils must be detoxified by our liver and kidneys. Therefore, it is imperative that you research an oil's properties before use to make sure it is not contraindicated for your health. Essential oils can also be harmful to small children, the elderly, people with liver or kidney issues, pregnant women, and animals. In these cases, please seek the guidance of a qualified healthcare practitioner before using them.

HOW TO STORE ESSENTIAL OILS

› Always store essential oils in a cool, dark cabinet away from heat and light and out of the reach of children and pets.

› Store essential oils in dark colored glass, which allows them to last longer.

› Don't store essential oils with rubber-top droppers in the bottle because they can break down the rubber. Instead use a screw cap or the drop-by-drop reducers that come in small bottles.

GENERAL ESSENTIAL OIL SAFETY GUIDELINES

› Do not take essential oils internally. Teas or tinctures are the appropriate methods for ingesting aromatics.

› Never use essential oils undiluted on your body, and do not use them near the eyes or mucus membranes.

› If you have not used a particular oil before, perform a small patch test on your inner forearm or your back by applying a small quantity of diluted essential oil to the skin, then cover with a bandage. If you experience any irritation, wash immediately and do not use that oil. If no irritation occurs after 48 hours, it is safe to use on your skin.

The National Association for Holistic Aromatherapy has an excellent webpage on safety information: https://naha.org/explore-aromatherapy/safety. For more information, we suggest that you speak with a licensed aromatherapist, naturopath, or qualified healthcare practitioner to ensure essential oils are safe for your purposes before use. The book *Essential Oil Safety: A Guide for Health Care Professionals* (2nd ed.) by Robert Tisserand and Rodney Young is a wonderful resource if you are serious about using essential oils regularly. This text is considered the industry standard reference for essential oil safety.

Diluting Essential Oils for Body and Hair Care Formulations

Essential oils must be diluted for safe use, whether you plan to use them on their own in a neutral carrier oil or as ingredients in a finished product such as a massage oil, lotion, or aroma spray. Whichever dilution method you choose, the essential oil content should only account for 0.5 to 2 percent of the total blend. This equates to three to twelve drops per ounce of finished product. This dilution takes into consideration that creams, lotions, serums, and other products are often applied liberally, frequently, and to large portions of the body and that fragrance is usually a secondary concern to a formulation's primary function of moisturizing and smoothing.

Perfumes containing essential oils are a bit different. Since these formulations are generally applied sparingly and to localized areas, you may choose to use a higher proportion, up to 5 percent, to allow your aroma blends to shine.

For easier versions of all this math, use this dilution chart.

Carrier	To achieve	
	1 percent essential oil	2 percent essential oil
5 ml	1 drop	2 drops
10 ml	2 drops	4 drops
½ oz	3 drops	6 drops
1 oz	6 drops	12 drops
2 oz	12 drops	¼ tsp
4 oz	¼ tsp	½ tsp
6 oz	36 drops	¾ tsp
8 oz	½ tsp	1 tsp
16 oz	1 tsp	2 tsp

Note: A handy dilution calculator is also available at https://blog.mountainroseherbs.com/ little-book-of-body-care-dilution

Essential Oil Conversion Chart

The potent nature of essential oils often means that only tiny volumes are needed, so it makes sense to measure amounts in drops. For those looking to make larger batches, however, counting out several hundred drops of liquid is simply not practical, and drops are also not very reliable on a larger scale. If you've ever wondered how to convert drops into standardized units like milliliters, teaspoons, and ounces, you aren't alone! We've put together this helpful essential oil conversion chart to make measuring and scaling your essential oil recipes faster, easier, and more accurate.

Note: An easy conversion calculator is also available at https://blog.mountainroseherbs.com/ little-book-of-body-care-conversion

Drops	Milliliters	Teaspoons	Tablespoons	Ounces
10	½			
20	1			
25	1¼	¼		
50	2½	½		
100	5	1		
	10	2		
	15	3	1	½
	30	6	2	1
	60	12	4	2
	120	24	8	4
	240	48 ½	16	8
	480	97 ½	32	16

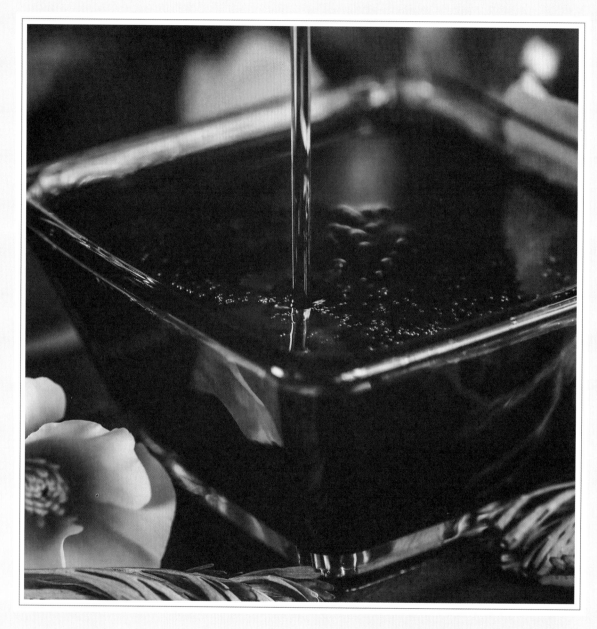

Understanding the differences in carrier oils will help you create recipes that best match your skin and hair care goals.

Guide to
Carrier Oils

Carrier oils are commonly pressed from the seeds, nuts, kernels, or fruits of plants. They range in color and scent depending on the plant and refinement process. Carrier oils with more unsaturated fats (like olive oil and almond oil) will pour easily and remain liquid at room temperature, whereas those with more saturated fats (like coconut oil) will be solid at room temperature. Carrier oils may be used alone or blended with other oils and are an integral component in many DIY body and hair care formulations. They are also used to safely dilute pure essential oils.

It is important to purchase carrier oils from a trustworthy source to ensure the best quality and that they are ethically sourced. Look for organic oils whenever possible, and choose pure oils that are cold pressed or expeller pressed. Avoid oils that have been extracted or refined using solvents or other chemicals. There are many excellent unrefined oils, as well as options that have been physically refined rather than chemically refined to remove color, strong scents, or fats so the oil doesn't separate in the cold.

Favorite Carrier Oils

Organic avocado oil (*Persea americana*) This emollient, highly permeating oil has an impressive nutritional profile that makes it an ideal ingredient for skin care recipes intended for dry, dehydrated, and mature skin, as well as nourishing, moisturizing hair care formulations. Avocado oil does add a slightly grassy aroma to skin care products, so keep this in mind when creating formulations.

Organic jojoba oil (*Simmondsia chinensis*) This product is actually a liquid wax, which gives jojoba oil it a stable shelf life. Structurally it resembles sebum, the oil that our skin naturally produces. Because of this, we love it for moisturizing massage and body oils. Jojoba oil can be used as a single ingredient base and does not need to be blended with other oils. Additionally, jojoba will not affect the scent of a finished blend.

Organic olive oil (*Olea europaea*) This classic oil is most often used in massage oils and as a medium for herbal oil infusions. Olive oil can feel slightly greasy to the touch, but it provides emollient properties to a blend and long-lasting glide to massage oils. Olive oil does have a strong aroma that can affect your finished product, but don't let that deter you from using this wonderful carrier oil.

Organic rosehip seed oil (*Rosa* spp.) This oil is our favorite for mature and dry skin, and it makes a wonderful moisturizing ingredient for facial serums and lotions. Although rosehip seed oil needs to be blended with another carrier and should not be used as a single ingredient base, it could make up to 20 percent of your base blend. We recommend refrigeration of this delicate oil after opening to preserve its shelf life.

Organic sunflower oil (*Helianthus annuus*) This high-oleic oil absorbs well into the skin, making sunflower oil a wonderful single ingredient base for body oils and massage oils. It has a light aroma that will not overpower the scent of a blend.

Organic sweet almond oil (*Prunus dulcis*) This oil is a classic base for body oils, creams, lotions, and soap. We love sweet almond oil for its emollient and moisturizing properties, and it can be used as a stand-alone base. Although you may be able to smell some of its nutty aroma, it will not overpower the scent of a finished blend.

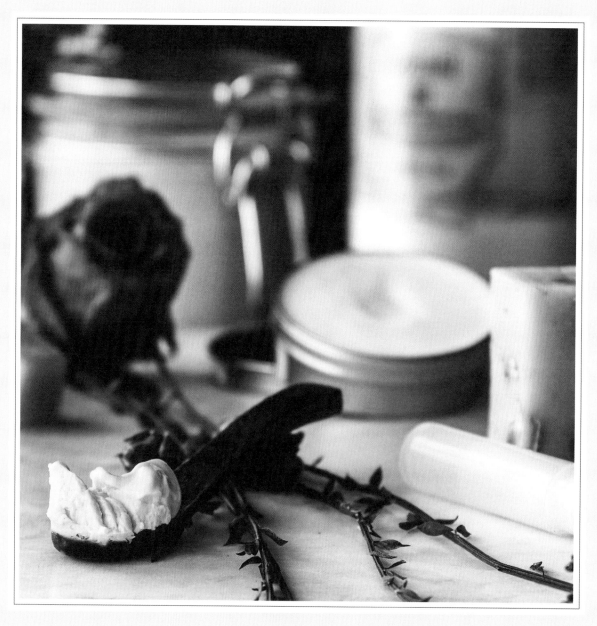

Knowing how to substitute ingredients appropriately is crucial when you've run out of something or want to replace an item in a recipe.

Guide to Substituting Ingredients in Body Care Recipes

The seemingly endless variety of recipes for body butters, skin oils, and other DIY personal care products is often inspiring, but it can also be overwhelming. This is further complicated by the fact that each of us is unique, with different sensitivities and preferences. In case you need or want to avoid a particular ingredient for any such reason, we have some tips to help you make appropriate ingredient substitutions and adapt these body care recipes to your needs.

First and foremost, be sure that your ingredients are 100 percent pure to avoid any recipe complications, as many companies carry oils that are preblended. This happens often with popular oils such as argan or jojoba. If an oil is blended, it should be clearly labeled with an ingredient list.

Also, if your substitution doesn't work out the way you wanted it to, don't despair. Many of the DIY body care recipes in this book can be gently melted down again to add more oil if they are too hard or butter or wax if they need more stability.

Breaking Down Basic Substitutions

Formulations are designed to be applied in certain ways and to impart certain benefits. A facial moisturizer, for instance, is intended to lightly nourish delicate skin without heaviness. A dense body butter, on the other hand, uses humectants like beeswax to help attract and retain moisture from the air and offer a protective layer of lasting hydration to extra-dry areas.

No one knows your skin better than you do. Experimentation is often the best way to become familiar with the ingredients that will be ideal for you. Making small test batches will save you time and money in the long run by helping determine if a recipe gives you the results you want. Happily, there are some general guidelines that may help to make your trial-and-error process more efficient.

To make ingredient substitutions that preserve the general character and function of a formulation, we focus on three main ingredient characteristics: consistency, absorption rate, and skin type compatibility.

Substituting by consistency

The easiest rule for substituting oils or butters is to match the consistency. When trading one ingredient for another, make sure it is close to the same texture and state at room temperature and when applied to skin. From a consistency perspective, oils that are liquid at room temperature can be used interchangeably.

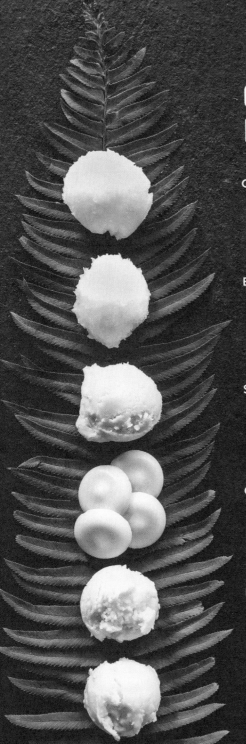

OILS & BUTTERS
BY CONSISTENCY

COCONUT OIL

softest

BABASSU OIL

SHEA BUTTER

COCOA BUTTER

KOKUM BUTTER

hardest

MANGO BUTTER

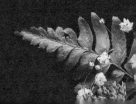

Substituting by absorption rate

Different oils are absorbed by the skin at different rates, which affects how heavy or light the formulation feels. If a formulation calls for a light facial oil like argan or camellia oil, castor oil will not make a pleasant substitution. So, if you need to substitute one oil for another and your goal is to have a finished product that is comparable to the original recipe, it is important to choose an oil with a similar absorption rate.

On the other hand, if you want the final product to be somewhat different to customize it to your needs, you can substitute for an ingredient with a different absorption profile. For instance, if a moisturizer recipe uses jojoba oil and rosehip seed oil and you want a denser moisturizer, you might replace the quick-absorbing rosehip seed oil with a medium-absorbing one like almond oil. With a few tweaks, you can make any recipe completely your own!

Keep in mind, matching absorption rates can be a bit tricky because we are each unique and different skin types react to oils differently. This is why we also must consider substituting by skin type.

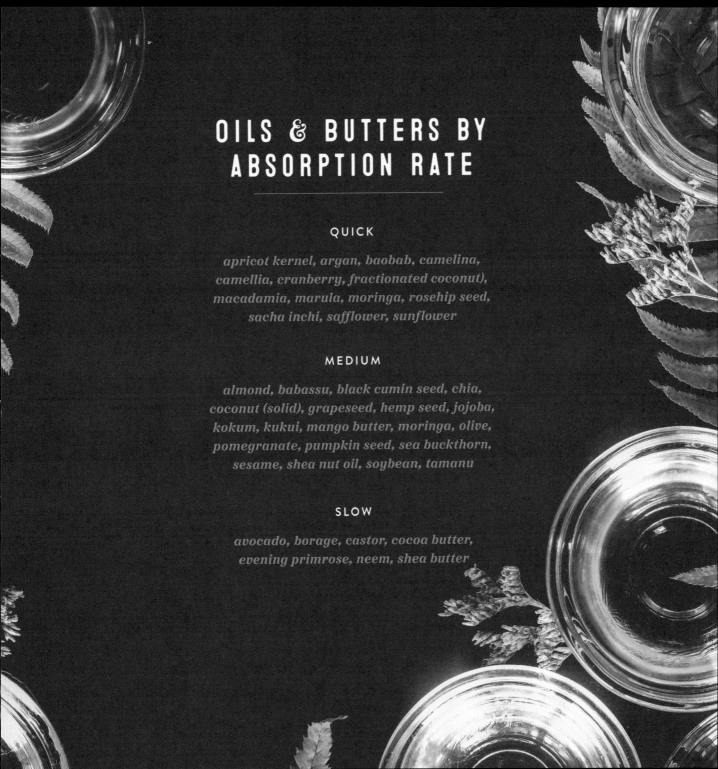

OILS & BUTTERS BY ABSORPTION RATE

QUICK

apricot kernel, argan, baobab, camelina, camellia, cranberry, fractionated coconut), macadamia, marula, moringa, rosehip seed, sacha inchi, safflower, sunflower

MEDIUM

almond, babassu, black cumin seed, chia, coconut (solid), grapeseed, hemp seed, jojoba, kokum, kukui, mango butter, moringa, olive, pomegranate, pumpkin seed, sea buckthorn, sesame, shea nut oil, soybean, tamanu

SLOW

avocado, borage, castor, cocoa butter, evening primrose, neem, shea butter

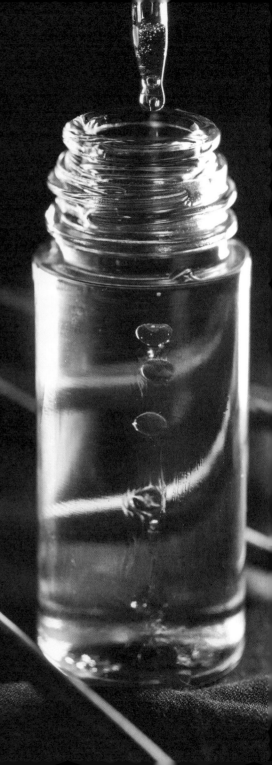

OILS & BUTTERS BY SKIN TYPE

NONCOMEDOGENIC

apricot kernel, argan, black cumin seed, borage, camellia, castor, grapeseed, hazelnut, hemp, jojoba, olive, pomegranate, pumpkin, rosehip, safflower, tamanu

FOR SENSITIVE OR MATURE SKIN

argan, camellia, jojoba, safflower, sea buckthorn, sesame, sunflower

FOR DRY SKIN

almond, argan, avocado, cranberry, hemp, jojoba, macadamia, marula, neem, shea oil

FOR OILY SKIN

argan, borage, castor, evening primrose, jojoba, rosehip

Substituting by skin type

Our skin's needs vary and change over time, affected by our genes, our age, our diet and exercise, the environment we live in, the weather, and more. Some oils are better suited to different skin types.

Noncomedogenic oils Skin that is prone to clogged pores and occasional cystic acne can benefit from moisturizers based on noncomedogenic ingredients. Most of these oils absorb at quick or medium rates and include favorites like argan, rosehip seed, pomegranate, and jojoba.

Oils for sensitive or mature skin When a delicate touch is in order, try formulating your products with ingredients like camellia, sea buckthorn, and sesame oils (a favorite for baby massage).

Oils for dry skin When you need a lasting hydration boost, opt for a deeply nourishing oils like avocado, cranberry, or marula.

Oils for oily skin Ingredients like castor, evening primrose, and borage can deliver nutrients to oily and combination skin without leaving extra shine behind.

Substituting for beeswax

Beeswax has been a common body care staple since ancient times, but there are other ingredients you can use in its place, if needed. Whether you're looking for a vegan option in a traditional recipe or you need to avoid an allergen, organic carnauba wax can be a good choice.

Note, however, that carnauba wax is much harder than beeswax, so we recommend replacing the required amount of beeswax with a mix of half carnauba wax, half soft plant oil (such as coconut oil). This combination works well for making plant-based salves, lip balms, and even candles!

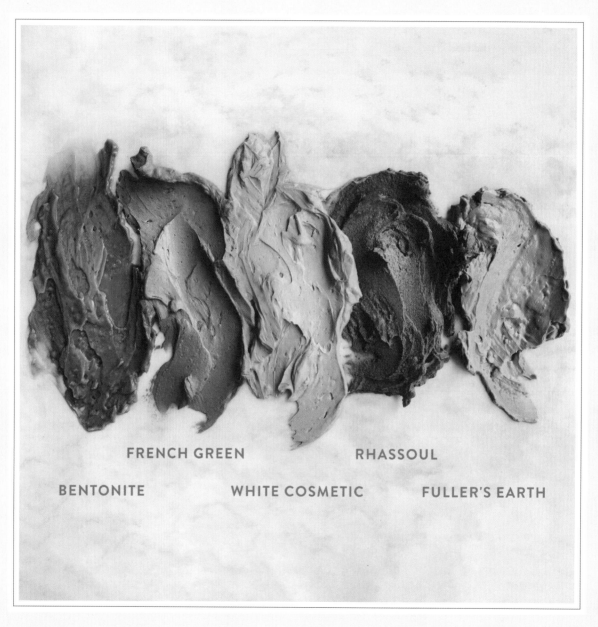

FRENCH GREEN   RHASSOUL

BENTONITE   WHITE COSMETIC   FULLER'S EARTH

Different cosmetic clays have a variety of drawing abilities.

Guide to Types of Cosmetic Clay and Their Uses

Cosmetic clays have long been known to provide beneficial properties for all kinds of skin types. They are commonly used in facial masks, dry shampoos, soaps, and body powders. Clays can also be added to the bath for a mineral-infused soak.

There are so many kinds of cosmetic clays available today, it can be difficult to choose the one that is right for you. All clays will draw oil from the skin, though some have stronger drawing abilities than others. For instance, those who tend to have drier skin may find that white cosmetic clay is preferable. People with oilier skin, on the other hand, might choose Fuller's earth clay.

Favorite Cosmetic Clays

BENTONITE CLAY

Sodium bentonite clay is composed of volcanic ash sediments that have been weathered over a long period of time. Bentonite clay is known for its absorbing properties, as it acts like a sponge when mixed with water. This clay is very popular for facial masks, foot baths, or bath soaking blends.

Dry characteristics When dry, bentonite clay has a neutral scent and a pale, off-white color. The texture is slightly grainy, but it smooths out when pressed between the fingers. While it does leave something of a powdery coating behind when brushed off, the dry clay does not stick to skin too much.

Wet characteristics When wet, the clay paste is off-white with a smooth consistency. If liquid is added in too slowly, clumps will form; the use of a whisk is helpful for keeping a smooth consistency.

This wet clay spreads smoothly on skin, and its thick texture is reminiscent of cooked oatmeal.

FRENCH GREEN CLAY

Although this fine-textured clay can be found in a variety of places around the globe, French green clay is so named because some of the first recorded deposits were in France. It gets its verdant color from decomposed plant matter. Many people find French green clay to be helpful for occasional blemishes, and it is generally used by those with average to oily skin.

Dry characteristics Dry French green clay has a neutral earthy aroma and pale green color. Although it has a fine texture, this clay does not puff (create a cloud of fine dust) out of the bag and has a slight graininess.

Wet characteristics The wet paste of French green clay has a somewhat darker hue and tends to have a slight lumpiness. Be sure to mix slowly and thoroughly with a whisk when adding liquid for smoother clay preparations. The texture can be a bit grainy when applied to the skin and has a thin consistency when spread out.

FULLER'S EARTH CLAY

Fuller's earth clay has very strong oil absorbing abilities, so it is recommended for those with very oily skin. This clay is also helpful in stain removal and has mild natural bleaching properties.

Dry characteristics The dry clay has a lightly earthy scent and an off-white to greenish and tan color. The texture is fine and powdery. It is also very lightweight, so watch out—it can get everywhere!

Wet characteristics Fuller's earth clay is very smooth and easy to mix with liquids. The color is dark gray to dark tan, and it retains a fairly thick consistency when wet.

RHASSOUL CLAY

Rhassoul clay is a fine, red-colored clay from Morocco that has been used for centuries in natural skin care. While it will still absorb oils from the skin, it is much gentler than many other clays and is typically recommended for more sensitive or mature skin types.

Dry characteristics When dry, Rhassoul clay has a light reddish-brown color and a fine texture; its slight grain feels similar to that of French green clay. However, unlike French clay, its lightness gives it a tendency to slightly puff out of an opened bag.

Wet characteristics Rhassoul clay mixes easily with water to create a darker, red-brown paste without lumps. It still retains a slight graininess, though this goes away as the clay absorbs water. It's easy to smooth onto skin and has a thin consistency when spread out.

WHITE COSMETIC CLAY

White cosmetic clay, also known as Kaolin clay, is not as absorbent as other clays, making it appropriate for skin that tends to be drier or more sensitive. Often, this clay is found as an ingredient in mineral makeup.

Dry characteristics White cosmetic clay has a neutral scent and a light tan color that can vary to off-white. The texture is very fine and soft, and it will coat skin with a thin powdery layer when handled.

Wet characteristics When liquid is added, white cosmetic clay takes on a much darker tan color. The texture remains fine and mixes easily with water, and it is smooth and grit-free.

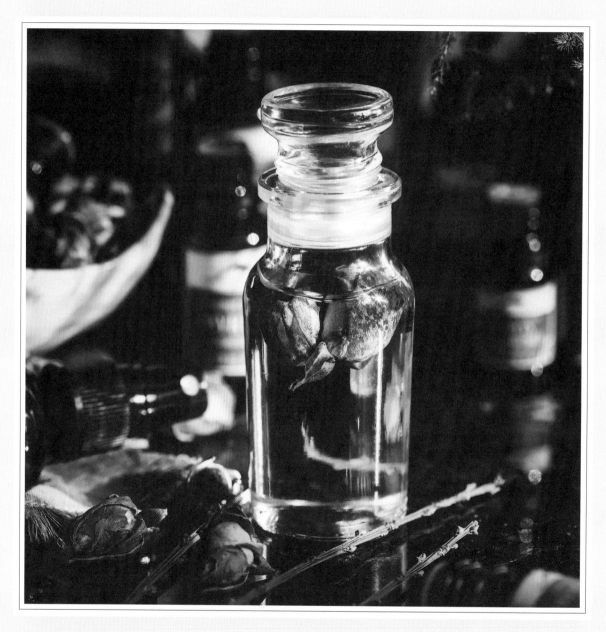

*For water-based products, it's often better
to simply make small batches as needed.*

Guide to Preserving Handcrafted & Natural Body Care Products

Following proper sterilization practices and working with beginner-friendly recipes allows you to get started on hair and body care crafting recipes that do not require advanced understanding about preservation methods. The following practices are fundamental to creating and storing herbal body care products safely.

Keep it clean Use clean, sterilized jars and containers. If you are recycling containers, make sure they have been put through a dishwasher or are washed well with soap and hot water. If you are purchasing new tins, jars, or bottles, it's still a good idea to wash them before use. We like to add a bit of white vinegar for extra measure and allow the containers to dry completely before use. Make sure there are no bits of food or other particles in the containers before you use them. This goes for infusion jars too—bacteria and moisture can quickly make oils go rancid.

Consider having designated equipment Having a special pot that you use only for DIY crafting, along with other tools like a blender or immersion blender, utensils, and glass measuring bowls that are committed only to body care products helps keep a separation between food prep and lotion prep.

Thoroughly strain out plant material Straining as much plant material as possible from your infusions before storing will help them to last longer.

When making water-based recipes, take extra precautions Water-based recipes include those with hydrosols, aloe vera gel, witch hazel extract, tea or water infusion, and vegetable glycerin. To eliminate possible contaminants, always use distilled water or boil water and allow it to cool prior to including it in recipes. Storing hydrosols, witch hazel extract, and aloe vera gel in the refrigerator can also help extend their shelf life.

Use antioxidants to extend shelf life Oxidation is what happens when exposure to air or oxygen starts to compromise the ingredients, especially carrier oils. Antioxidants like vitamin E oil and rosemary antioxidant oil are good examples of natural stabilizers that help to slow oxidation in vulnerable ingredients. We often include these in homemade serums, massage oils, and lip gloss recipes to help preserve the integrity of the finished product. They are typically added to recipes after the use of direct heat.

Use alcohol as a preservative in water-based formulations You can include alcohol extracts or tinctures to a recipe to help with preservation and add botanical goodness. Just plain organic alcohol like vodka works too! Keep in mind that alcohol doesn't mix well with all fats, so its use should be limited to water-based body care products.

Make small batches As a rule, water-based creations will have a much shorter shelf life than oil- or butter-based ones, because water breeds life! For water-based products like hair rinses, it's often better to simply make small batches as needed. This has the added benefit of ensuring that you are using the freshest ingredients in your daily routine.

Properly store your creations A good rule is to store your DIY body care products out of direct light and where they will not be subject to temperature fluctuations. Infused oils, butters, and beeswax are best stored in cool, dry places. You will sometimes see us recommend that a finished product be stored in a cobalt or amber bottle or jar rather than a clear container. The dark color helps keep out strong light that can speed up deterioration. Some creations, especially water-based ones, are best stored in the refrigerator.

Wash your hands before use Putting dirty hands into jars of salve or lotion can introduce bacteria and shorten the product's shelf life. It's a good idea to give your hands/fingers a quick wash and dry before dipping. For oils, consider using a bottle with a flip top or pump to cut down on the chances of introducing bacteria.

Close container lids tightly between uses Clean, snug lids keep out light and oxygen.

Guide to Measurement Conversions

SMALL MEASUREMENTS

Milliliters	Teaspoons	Tablespoons
2½	½	
5	1	
15	3	1

DRY VOLUMES

Ounces	Tablespoons	Cups
1	2	⅛
2	4	¼
4	8	½
8	16	1
16	32	2

General Kitchen Conversions

DRY MEASUREMENTS

Cups	Teaspoons	Tablespoons
	3	1
⅛	6	2
¼	12	4
½	24	8
¾	36	12
1	48	16

Product-Specific Conversions

COCOA BUTTER WAFERS

1 tsp	5 grams	2 wafers
1 Tbsp	12 grams	5 wafers

BEESWAX PASTILLES

1 tsp	3 grams
1 Tbsp	9 grams

LIQUID VOLUMES AND MEASUREMENTS

Milliliters	Teaspoons	Tablespoons	Fluid Ounces	Cups	Pints	Quarts	Gallons
59	12	4	2	¼			
118	24	8	4	½			
237	48	16	8	1	½	¼	
473	96	32	16	2	1	½	
			32	4	2	1	¼
			64	8	4	2	½
			128	16	8	4	1

US to Metric Conversions

Cups	Mililiters	Fl Ounces
	30	1
¼	59	
⅓	79	
½	119	
⅔	158	
¾	178	
1	237	

The Folk Method of Measuring in Parts

Back in the day, herbalists did not have exact measuring implements, so they learned to cook and formulate using the tools at hand: a teacup, a wooden spoon, a handful. By using those same tools, early herbalists could create and reproduce consistent recipes or formulations and could then easily share them with others. This convenient, universal measuring system made it possible to pass herbal wisdom down through the generations.

Measuring in parts is still a remarkably useful skill in creating herbal formulations—as well as culinary recipes—because it works with ratios, which makes it easy to scale a recipe up or down in size.

A part doesn't have to be as random as your grandma's soup spoon; it can be a precise measurement. So, for instance, if a recipe is one part wax to four parts carrier oil, each of those parts might be 1 Tablespoon or 1 ounce or 1 cup. If you know the ratio, you can measure by volume or by weight. In this example, if you were using ¼ cup (one part) of beeswax, you would need approximately 1 cup (four parts) of carrier oil. Alternatively, if you were using ¼ pound (one part) of beeswax, you would need approximately 1 pound (four parts) of carrier oil.

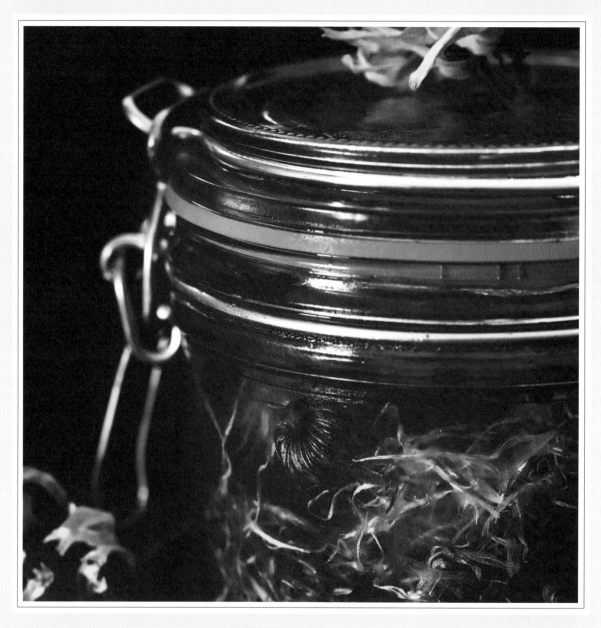

Infused oils act as a vehicle to deliver beneficial constituents from the plant to your skin.

Guide to Making Herb-Infused Oils for Body Care

The world of herbalism is vast in a way that can seem daunting for those new to the botanical arts. That's why when we're trying to help friends get started in herbs without overwhelming them, we often recommend one of our favorite herbalism projects for beginners: making herb-infused oils. Simply infusing a carrier oil with herbs will transform it into a versatile ingredient. Herb-infused oils can be used to create salves, massage oils, lip balms, facial serums, hair treatments, body creams, soaps, and more!

Oil Infusing Basics

While most herbs can be infused either dried or fresh (with proper preparation), we usually recommend using dried herbs, especially for beginners. If you want to use fresh herbs, wilt them first for 12 hours to remove the moisture—too much water will cause the oil to go rancid. Next, cut the herbs into small pieces or crush with a mortar and pestle before adding them to a sterilized infusion container. Many different organic carrier oils may be used, however fractionated coconut oil (also sometimes called MCT coconut oil) and olive oil are popular and wise choices because they have long shelf lives and are suitable for many applications.

Herb-infused oils can turn rancid or grow mold, especially if the carrier oil used is not very shelf stable (such as rosehip seed oil) or if fresh herbs are used. For safety reasons, infused oils that exhibit any change in color, scent, or clarity should be discarded.

TIPS FOR SUCCESS

› Adding a preservative like vitamin E oil will help oils stay stable longer.
› When infused in oil, herbs such as annatto seed, spirulina, cocoa, and turmeric root may add color to soaps and other body care formulations.
› You may want to wear gloves when it comes time to strain a finished herb-infused oil. While you can use your bare hands, working with oils is a messy process, and certain herbs, like turmeric, may temporarily stain your hands and jewelry.
› Oil can be difficult to wash out of cheesecloth or muslin. Wash straining material in hot, soapy water or put it in the dishwasher to clean.
› Even after straining, fine herb sediment can make oil a bit gritty. If this bothers you, allow the oil to settle and then pour the clean infusion off the top of the grit. You can also strain it again through a coffee filter; this is a slow-drip process and may require more than one coffee filter to strain all the oil.
› Herbs can be blended together for synergistic infusions. For example, hops flowers, lavender flowers, and chamomile flowers infused together in jojoba oil make a wonderful relaxing massage oil blend. Mix and match to suit your needs!

Three Methods of Infusing Oil with Herbs

There are several ways to infuse oils. The easiest option is the folk (or simplers) method, which relies on the sun to naturally infuse oil with herbal properties. If you're short on time, you can instead use a heat infusion method. We will also explain an alcohol intermediary method for creating very shelf-stable oil infusions perfect for salves and other body care formulations.

FOLK METHOD FOR SOLAR-INFUSED OILS

Use the sun to naturally infuse oil with the goodness of organic herbs! Herb-infused oils made using this method can be used for both culinary and body care recipes. For example, rosemary-infused olive oil makes both an excellent hydrating hair mask and a flavorful salad dressing base. For food purposes, just be sure that the oil and the herb(s) you choose are both tasty and safe to eat.

DIRECTIONS

1. Place the herbs in a clean, dry glass jar. Leave at least 2 to 3 inches of open space above the herbs to cover with oil and to allow for any swelling that may occur as the herbs soak up the oil. The amount of herbs you use will depend on the size of the jar.

2. Fill the remaining space in the jar with your oil of choice, making sure to cover the herbs by at least 1 inch or more.

3. Cap the jar tightly and shake well.

4. Place the jar on a sunny, warm windowsill and shake once or more per day for 2 to 3 weeks. If the herbs emerge above the surface of the oil at any point while infusing, pour more oil on top to ensure they remain covered.

5. Strain the herbs out of the oil through cheesecloth or a fine mesh strainer. Make sure to squeeze out as much of the precious oil as possible. Compost or discard the herbs.

6. Pour the herb-infused oil into a sterilized glass jar.

7. *Optional:* To prolong the shelf life of oils to be used topically (not for culinary uses), add vitamin E oil at a concentration of up to 1 percent. For example, add 1 teaspoon of vitamin E oil to 16 fluid ounces of herb-infused oil. Cap the jar and swirl to blend in the vitamin E oil.

8. Label the jar with the date and ingredient list including herbs, carrier oil, and optional vitamin E if used.

9. Store in a cool, dark place. Oils will keep for up to 1 year. Be sure to check them regularly for any signs of spoilage.

TIPS

Some herbalists prefer to cover the jar while in the window with a brown paper bag to keep the herbs away from direct sunlight.

It is common to have some pieces of herbs that float in the oil after saturation. If these float to the top where they are exposed to air and start to mold or decay, simply skim them off and discard them.

QUICK METHOD FOR HEAT-INFUSED OILS

The quick method utilizing heat is sometimes necessary when you need herb-infused oils but you don't have 2 to 3 weeks to wait. This method must be done carefully, however, because it is easy to overheat the herbs. As with the folk method, heat-infused oils can be used in both culinary and topical preparations, as long as both the oil and the herb(s) you choose are suitable to ingest.

DIRECTIONS

1. Place the herbs in a crock-pot, double boiler, or electric yogurt maker, and cover with your carrier oil of choice, making sure to add enough oil to cover the herbs by at least 1 to 2 inches. The amount of herbs you use will depend on the size of the vessel you are putting them in.

2. Gently heat at a very low temperature (preferably between 100°F and 140°F) for 1 to 5 hours. Some people recommend heating the oil for 48 to 72 hours at a controlled temperature of 100°F. Turn off the heat and allow to cool.

3. Strain the herbs out of the oil through cheesecloth or a fine mesh strainer. Make sure to squeeze out as much of the precious oil as possible. Compost or discard the herbs.

4. Pour the herb-infused oil into a sterilized glass jar.

5. *Optional*: To prolong the shelf life of oils to be used topically (not for culinary uses), add vitamin E oil at a concentration of up to 1 percent. For example, add 1 teaspoon of vitamin E oil to 16 ounces of herb-infused oil. Cap the jar and swirl to blend in the vitamin E oil.

6. Label the jar with the date and ingredient list including herbs, carrier oil, and optional vitamin E if used.

7. Store in a cool, dark place. Infused oils will keep for up to 1 year. Be sure to check them regularly for any signs of spoilage.

ALCOHOL INTERMEDIARY METHOD FOR TOPICAL HERB-INFUSED OILS

The alcohol and grinding in this method help to extract the maximum amount of goodness from botanicals, yielding oils of exceptional color and potency. This method also produces herb-infused oils that are much less prone to contamination than those infused using either the folk or heat infusion methods. However, oils infused in this way are *not* suitable for culinary use. Although most of the alcohol evaporates, a detectable and unpleasant taste will remain. The alcohol intermediary method requires 24 hours to complete and should only be used with dried herbs.

DIRECTIONS

1. Weigh out approximately 1 ounce of dried organic herb(s).

2. Using a coffee grinder, bullet grinder, or blender, grind the herbs until coarse, but not too fine (or it will be difficult to strain later).

3. Transfer the ground herbs into a clean jar with a tight-fitting lid.

4. Add 1 Tablespoon of 190-proof ethanol to the jar with the ground herbs.

5. Use a fork to work the herbs and alcohol together or put the lid on and shake to disperse the alcohol through the herb material—it should be the consistency of nice soil or damp beach sand.

6. Set aside for at least 24 hours to allow the herbs to macerate in the alcohol.

7. Put the damp herb material into a blender.

8. Add approximately 1 cup of carrier oil of choice. Add more as necessary to cover well and ensure the herbs are moving around in the blender.

9. Blend on high until the plant material is fully incorporated.

10. Place a good-sized mesh strainer over a bowl or large glass measuring cup. Line the strainer with cheesecloth or fine muslin.

11. Pour the herb-infused oil into the lined strainer and allow it to drain. Use the cheesecloth or muslin to squeeze out as much of the oil as possible from the herbs.

12. Pour the strained oil into a sterilized glass jar.

13. *Optional*: Add vitamin E oil at a concentration of up to 1 percent to prolong the oil's shelf life.

14. Label the jar with the date and ingredient list including herbs, carrier oil, and vitamin E if used.

15. Store in a cool, dark place. Oils will keep for up to 1 year. Be sure to check them regularly for any signs of spoilage.

TIPS

A measuring shot glass works great for getting accurate measurements of small quantities of alcohol. One shot equals 2 Tablespoons.

You can perform all of these steps in a blender with an airtight lid. Grind the herbs in the blender, then add the alcohol, mix as directed above, put the lid on tightly, and let the mixture sit for 24 hours right in the blender.

Some fluffy herbs like calendula won't grind well in large batches, so grind these in smaller quantities to get a good consistency.

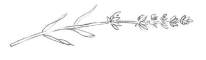

Natural Botanical Hair Care

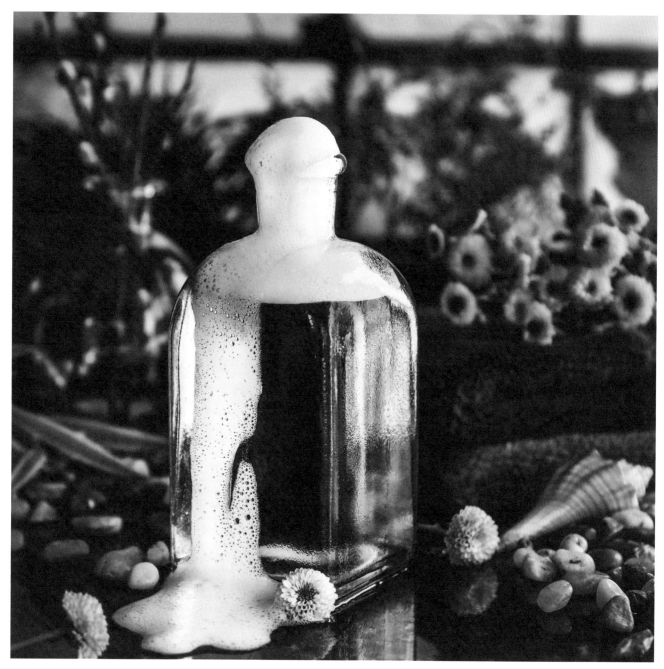

Making concentrates is a safe way to craft water-based recipes without having to worry about preservatives.

LIQUID SHAMPOO CONCENTRATE

Makes enough for 8 washes of medium-length hair

Keeping a natural liquid shampoo concentrate on hand is an easy way to ditch the synthetic additives and plastic packaging of store-bought shampoos. Plus, it lets you customize the scent of your homemade shampoo on a whim. Just mix with water anytime you're ready to shampoo.

INGREDIENTS

⅓ cup + 1 teaspoon liquid castile soap

20 to 60 drops organic lavender essential oil

¼ teaspoon organic rosemary-infused carrier oil (prepare ahead)

DIRECTIONS

1. Combine the ingredients in a bottle with an airtight lid.

2. Cap the bottle and roll it between your hands to blend.

3. Store in a cool dark place between uses. This concentrate is shelf stable for 1 month.

TO USE

1. Mix 3 parts water and 1 part base mixture in a container (1 teaspoon of the concentrate works well for medium-length hair).

2. Gently mix or shake well and apply to your hair. Massage into the scalp and rinse thoroughly.

3. Follow up with a conditioner, if you choose.

TIPS

Because there is no preservative in this mixture, we recommended that you do not mix it with water ahead of time. It will not be shelf stable.

Customize this recipe to your own preferences by changing the essential oil, herb-infused oil, or water for an herbal infusion of choice.

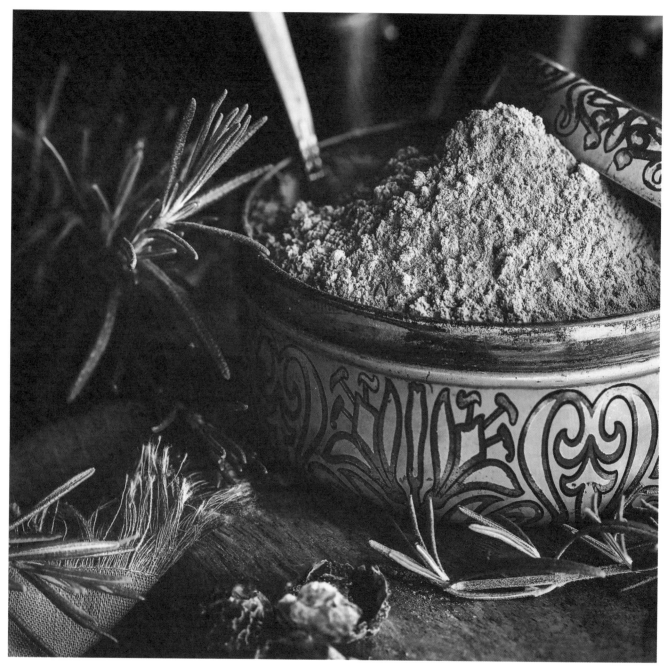

*This shampoo powder is a natural cleanser that's washed
out of the hair with water, like a standard shampoo.*

SHAMPOO POWDER

Makes about ½ cup

Although they sound the same, soap pod (*Acacia concinna*) and soap nut (*Sapindus trifoliatus*) are different botanicals. As well as being effective, they are good alternatives for people with skin conditions, sensitive skin, or chemical sensitivity.

INGREDIENTS

4 Tablespoons soap pod powder (also known as shikakai)

1 Tablespoon soap nut powder

1 Tablespoon organic amla powder

2 teaspoons organic fenugreek powder

2 teaspoons organic rosemary powder

DIRECTIONS

1. Thoroughly stir together all the powders.

2. When ready to use, mix 2 Tablespoons of the powder blend with enough water to make a watery paste.

3. Starting at your roots and working your way down, massage the paste into your hair.

4. Rinse completely and follow with a conditioner of your choice.

TIPS

If you cannot find soap nut powder, you can blend the deseeded shells in a blender or food processor to make powder.

Note that shampoo powder and dry shampoo are two different types of hair care products. Shampoo powder is a cleanser that is washed out of the hair with water, like a standard shampoo, while dry shampoo is used to lift oils from the hair in between washes and is not washed out after use. Dry shampoo is sometimes even used as a hair styling product to help add volume and lift.

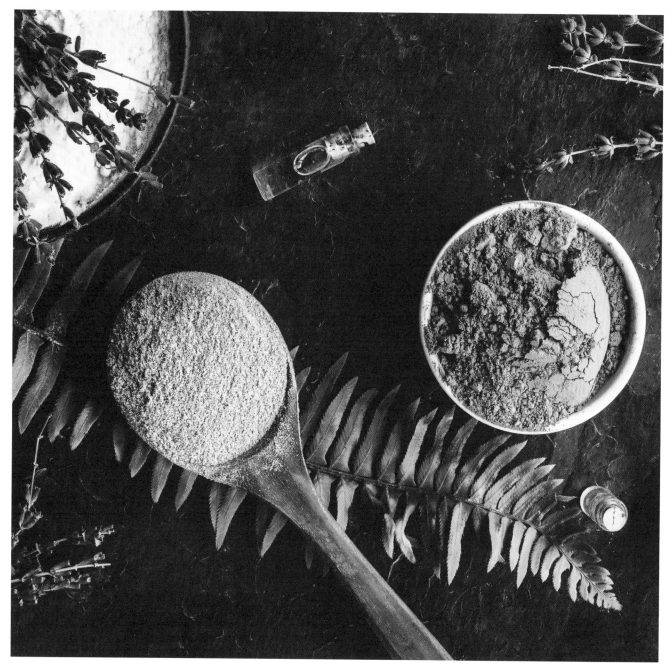

Dry shampoos are used between washings to lift oils from the hair and do not require washing out after use.

DRY SHAMPOO

Dry shampoos use powdered herbs, grains, and natural cosmetic clays that absorb excess oil, which are removed by brushing them out of the hair. These shampoos can also be a good option for folks who want to use regular shampoo less often, and they are also handy for camping trips and festivals. Depending on your hair color, choose the recipe that will work best for you.

DIRECTIONS

1. Mix all the ingredients together and stir well to combine.

2. Transfer the finished blend into a dry container and store away from moisture (to reduce clumping). Containers with shaker tops work well.

TO USE

1. Shake or sprinkle the powdered shampoo blend along the crown of the head, working through the scalp and hair to pick up any excess oils or debris.

2. Depending on the texture and thickness of your hair, either brush or shake your hair well to remove the excess powder. This is best done before you get dressed so you don't end up with powder residue on your clothes; you can also drape your shoulders with a towel to keep the powder off your clothes.

3. Use as necessary between washings.

Lavender and Sweet Orange Shampoo Powder for Light Hair

Makes about 1 ⅛ cups powder

INGREDIENTS

½ cup organic arrowroot powder

½ cup French green cosmetic clay

1 Tablespoon organic oatstraw powder

1 Tablespoon organic lavender flower powder

1 Tablespoon organic chamomile powder

10 drops organic sweet orange essential oil

10 drops organic lavender essential oil

Rosemary Cacao Shampoo Powder for Dark Hair

Makes about 1 ¼ cups powder

INGREDIENTS

½ cup organic arrowroot powder

¼ cup baking soda

½ cup organic cacao powder or organic carob powder

1 Tablespoon organic rosemary powder

1 Tablespoon organic oatstraw powder

10 drops organic rosemary essential oil

10 drops organic bergamot essential oil

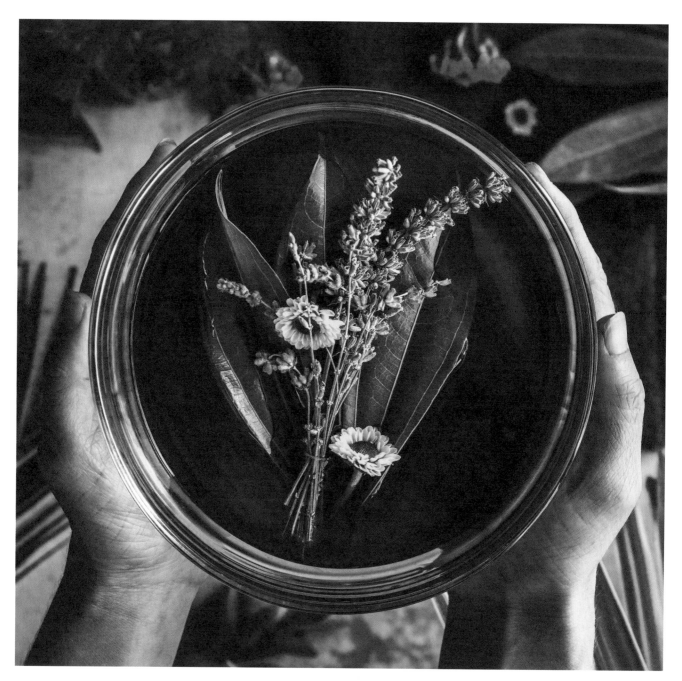

A mineral-rich nettle hair rinse yields the best result when used weekly.

NETTLE LAVENDER RINSE *for All Hair Types*

Makes about 2 ½ cups

Nettle infusions have long been used to promote healthy, shiny hair. Lavender essential oil helps normalize both dry and oily scalp conditions and is a nice choice for sensitive scalps. The two in combination make this formulation perfect for all hair colors and types.

INGREDIENTS

2 ½ cups organic nettle leaf tea, brewed strong (¼ cup dried herbs to 1 cup water)

5 drops organic lavender essential oil

1 Tablespoon baking soda

DIRECTIONS

1. To brew strong nettle leaf tea, gently simmer the appropriate amount of nettles in water for 10 to 15 minutes. Strain and compost the nettles.

2. Combine the tea, essential oil, and baking soda together in a glass jar. Cap the jar and shake to completely dissolve the baking soda and mix the ingredients.

3. Allow the mixture to cool to body temperature.

4. Pour over your dry hair or, alternatively, soak your hair in the mixture for at least 5 minutes. Massage your scalp gently using a circular motion.

5. Rinse thoroughly with clean running water.

6. You can follow the herbal rinse with an apple cider vinegar rinse for further conditioning and softening.

TIPS

If your hair feels dry and you want a little conditioning, add ⅛ teaspoon organic fractionated coconut oil to the recipe.

You'll get best results by using this rinse weekly.

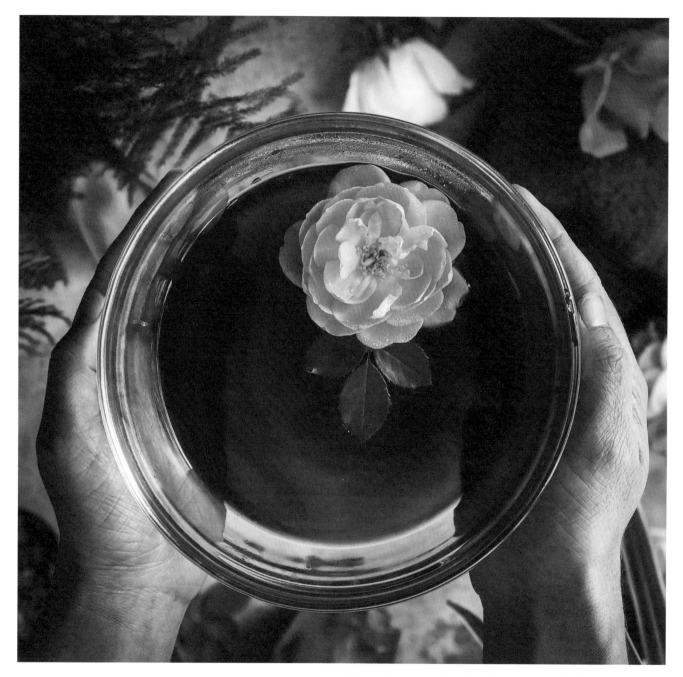

Chamomile is an excellent choice for rinses intended for lighter hair colors.

CHAMOMILE ROSE RINSE *for Light Hair*

The deep golden yellow produced by the chamomile flowers makes this a wonderful choice for light colored hair or to enhance natural highlights in darker hair.

INGREDIENTS

1 ½ cups organic chamomile tea, brewed strong (⅜ cup dried herbs to 1 ½ cups water)

1 cup organic rose petal or horsetail tea, brewed strong (¼ cup dried herbs to 1 cup water)

½ teaspoon baking soda

DIRECTIONS

1. To brew strong tea, gently simmer the appropriate amount of dried herbs in water for 10 to 15 minutes.

2. Strain the teas, and combine them with the baking soda in a glass jar. Cap the jar and shake to completely dissolve the baking soda and mix the ingredients.

3. Allow the mixture to cool to body temperature.

4. Pour over your dry hair or, alternatively, soak your hair in the mixture for at least 5 minutes. Massage your scalp gently using a circular motion.

5. Rinse out with clean running water.

6. You can follow the herbal rinse with an apple cider vinegar rinse for added conditioning and softening.

TIPS

If your hair feels dry and you want a little conditioning, you can add ⅛ teaspoon organic fractionated coconut oil to moisturize.

You'll get best results by using this rinse weekly.

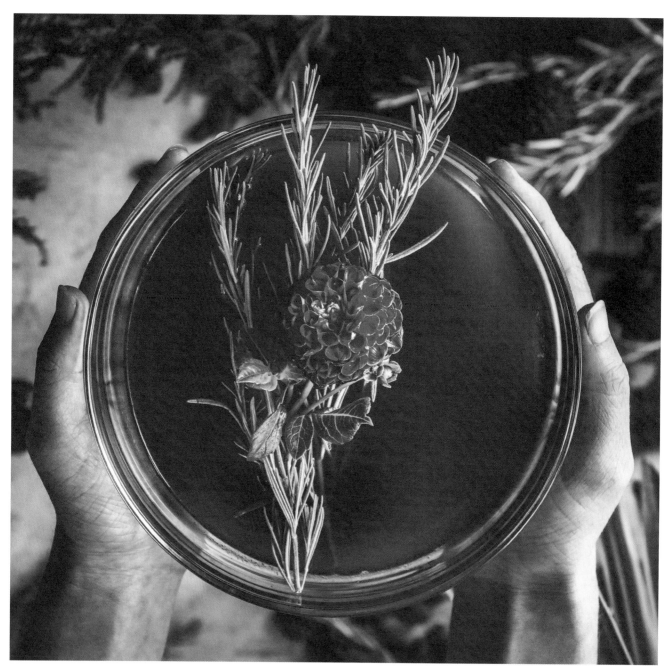

The natural fats in cacao help condition the scalp and are ideal for darker hair colors.

ROSEMARY CACAO RINSE *for Dark Hair*

Makes about 2 ½ cups

Rosemary helps stimulate scalp circulation and supports healthy follicles. The naturally conditioning cocoa butter fats found in cacao nibs will leave your hair feeling soft, and the chocolate-colored infusion is perfect for all shades of brown hair.

INGREDIENTS

1 ½ cups organic cacao tea, brewed strong (⅜ cup dried cacao nibs to 1 ½ cups water)

1 cup organic rosemary tea, brewed strong (¼ cup dried organic rosemary leaf to 1 cup water)

3 drops organic peppermint essential oil

½ teaspoon baking soda

DIRECTIONS

1. To brew strong tea, gently simmer the appropriate amount of dried herbs in water for 10 to 15 minutes.

2. Strain the teas, and combine them with the baking soda and essential oil in a glass jar. Cap the jar and shake to completely dissolve the baking soda and mix the ingredients.

3. Allow the mixture to cool to body temperature.

4. Pour over your dry hair or, alternatively, soak your hair in the mixture for at least 5 minutes. Massage your scalp gently using a circular motion.

5. Rinse out with clean running water.

6. You can follow the herbal rinse with an apple cider vinegar rinse for added conditioning and softening.

TIPS

If your hair feels dry and you want a little conditioning, you can add an additional ⅛ teaspoon organic fractionated coconut oil to moisturize.

You'll get best results by using this rinse weekly.

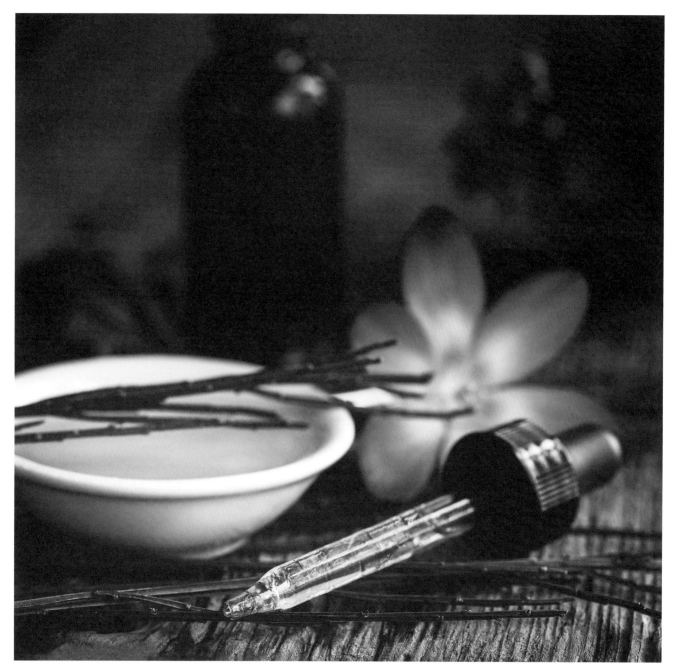

Leave-in conditioners hydrate your hair throughout the day and also help control frizz.

LEAVE-IN CONDITIONER
with ARGAN AND JOJOBA OILS

Makes about ⅛ cup

In those moments when a deeper moisturizing treatment is in order, this oil-based leave-in conditioner provides extra nourishment, helps tame wild fly-aways, softens brittle hair in dry temperatures, and protects your healthy mane.

INGREDIENTS

1 Tablespoon organic argan oil

1 Tablespoon organic jojoba oil

1 teaspoon organic pomegranate seed oil or organic castor oil (optional, use for dry/coarse hair)

5 drops organic rosemary essential oil

5 drops organic lavender essential oil

DIRECTIONS

1. Combine the carrier oils and essential oils in a glass bottle with a dropper.

2. Screw on the cap and roll the bottle between your palms to disperse the essential oils.

TO USE

1. For wet hair, place a couple of drops onto your fingertips and run them through your hair from midway to the ends. Brush through while your hair is still wet, and style as normal.

2. For dry hair, place a couple of drops onto your fingertips and run through your hair from midway to the ends. Avoid adding oils to your scalp directly, as this is where oil can build up.

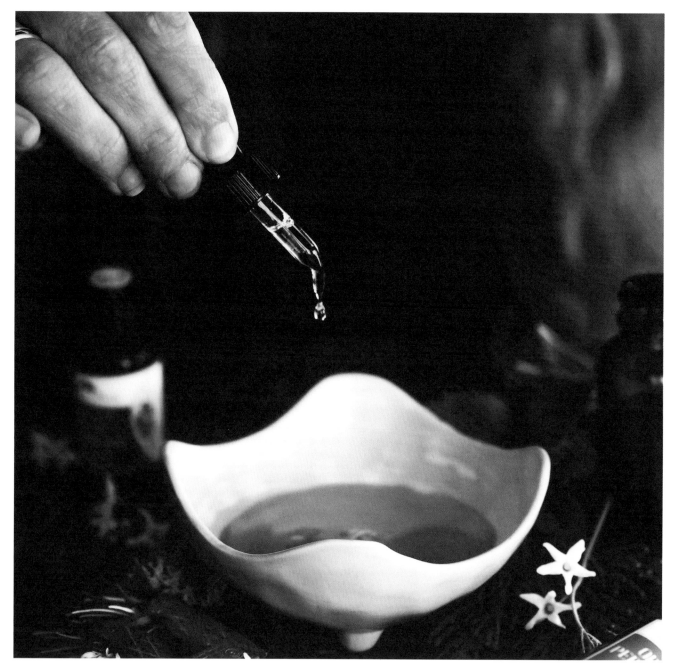

Hot oil treatments offer deeply penetrating and lasting support to the hair.

HOT OIL HAIR TREATMENT

Makes enough for 1 treatment of medium-length to long hair

Oil treatments are a great way to naturally condition, cleanse, and invigorate your hair and scalp. A few drops of this hot oil hair treatment can also help tame dry or wild-looking locks.

INGREDIENTS

1 Tablespoon organic coconut oil

1 Tablespoon organic argan oil

1 teaspoon organic neem oil or jojoba oil

1 teaspoon organic castor oil

7 drops organic cedarwood essential oil

4 drops vitamin E oil

DIRECTIONS

1. Add the coconut, argan, neem, and castor oils to a double boiler over medium heat and heat until warm.

2. Remove from the heat and thoroughly stir in the essential oil and vitamin E oil.

TO USE

1. Pour a little warm oil into your palm and massage it into your scalp and hair, working out any knots that may be present. Add as much as needed to thoroughly coat your hair and scalp.

2. Cover your head and hair with a plastic bag or shower cap and leave the oil in your hair for at least 20 to 30 minutes.

TIPS

Neem oil is not the most pleasant-smelling oil, but it is very good for the hair. If you prefer a more pleasant aromatic experience, opt for the jojoba oil.

Continued →

3. *Optional*: Heat deepens the oil's penetration and enhancesits benefits. Sit in the sunshine, next to a fire, or in a sauna. Alternatively, you can gently warm the oil to 100°F before you massage it into your hair and scalp. Then pull up your hair, cover it with a plastic bag or shower cap, and wrap it with a towel or wool cap to retain heat. Leave the oil in your hair, covered, for at least 1 hour.

4. Shampoo the oil out completely. Don't worry if your hair still feels a little oily after washing; it should absorb the residual oil as it dries.

5. Follow with conditioner if you choose.

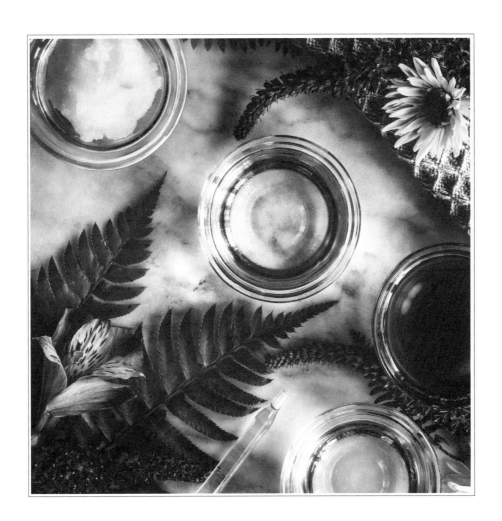

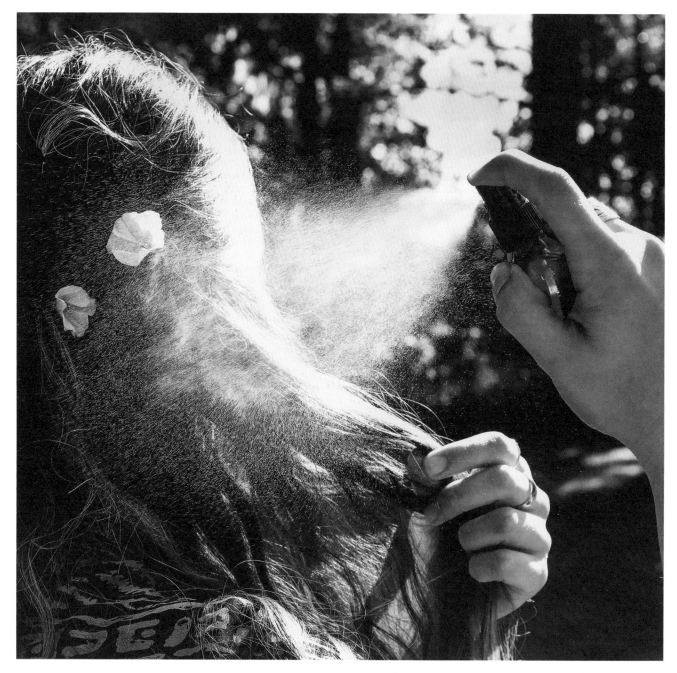

A simple salt hairspray is a great way to give your locks beachy waves.

BEACHY WAVES SALT HAIR SPRAY *with* ROSEMARY

Makes about 1 cup

Few things awaken our hair's inner mermaid like a salty dip and a sea breeze air-dry. When you can't get to the beach, salt sprays are an easy alternative. You can also add the fragrance and nourishing properties of pure essential oils and organic hydrosols to create gorgeous wavy hair that smells great!

INGREDIENTS

⅔ cup water

2 Tablespoons Epsom salt

½ teaspoon Himalayan pink salt

¼ cup organic peppermint hydrosol

1 teaspoon aloe vera gel

10 drops organic rosemary essential oil

DIRECTIONS

1. Add the water and salts to a medium saucepan. Heat the water until just warm enough to dissolve the salts.

2. Transfer the saltwater into an 8-ounce jar or glass bottle.

3 Allow the saltwater to cool to room temperature (15 to 20 minutes), then add the hydrosol, aloe vera gel, and essential oil. Cap and swirl to mix.

4. Store in a cool, dry place for up to 6 months. Decant part of the recipe into a 1- to 2-ounce glass bottle with a mister for ease of use.

TIPS

Shake well before each use.

Store the majority of your new salt spray in a glass jar or bottle. If you store all of it in the mister bottle, the salt will eventually clog the mister tip.

Folks with a variety of hair types can enjoy the benefits of salt spray. Those with wavy

Continued →

1. For natural, breezy waves, apply, scrunch, and let your hair air-dry.

2. Alternatively, blow dry with a diffuser attachment until your hair is almost, but not completely dry.

hair often find that a spritz or two helps give their natural curl more definition and less frizz, while straight-haired people use the spray to loosen up their locks. We recommend starting with less spray if your hair already tends to twist, or more if it likes to play it straight.

All salt sprays are a bit drying, so you'll get the best results when you apply to hair that already contains some of its natural oils. Avoid using directly after washing with a clarifying shampoo, or apply a conditioning cream or serum before spritzing with salt spray.

We find that this formulation works best when applied to damp (not soaking wet) hair. If applying after a shower, comb through your hair and let it dry partway before applying. Alternatively, spray your dry hair with plain water to moisten before using salt spray.

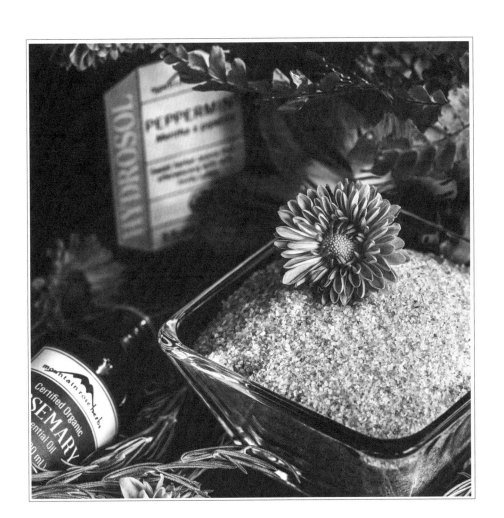

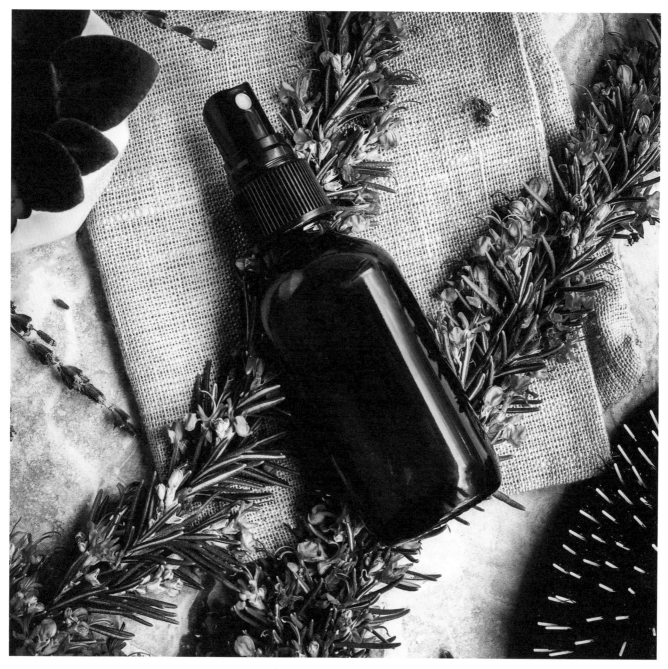

Aloe and marshmallow root help to remove tangles and provide protection from fly-aways.

DETANGLER & ANTI-FRIZZ SPRAY

Makes about 2 ¼ cups

When applied to wet hair, the mucilaginous quality of marshmallow root mixed with aloe vera gel coats, softens, and helps smooth out tangles. This spray will also help tame serious bedhead.

DIRECTIONS

1. Place the water and marshmallow root in a small saucepan and bring to a simmer. Simmer until reduced by half, which should take at least 30 minutes.

2. Strain out the liquid and compost the spent marshmallow root.

3. Allow the marshmallow tea mixture to cool.

4. Pour into an 8-ounce spray bottle, and add aloe vera gel, lavender essential oil, rosemary essential oil, and a carrier oil of choice.

5. Cap and shake to combine.

6. Keep refrigerated, and use it up within 1 to 2 weeks.

TO USE

1. Apply evenly over damp hair.

2. Gently brush though hair. Start at ends and work your way up.

3. Wash out and condition as normal.

INGREDIENTS

2 cups water

2 Tablespoons organic marshmallow root

2 Tablespoons aloe vera gel

20 drops organic lavender essential oil

10 drops organic rosemary essential oil

1 Tablespoon organic argan oil, organic jojoba oil, or organic avocado oil (optional)

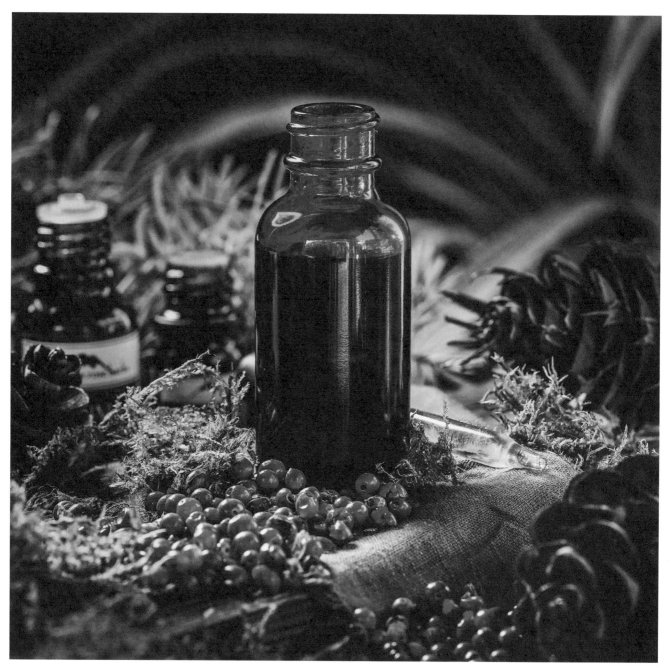

Beard oils condition facial hair and are also an excellent vehicle for fragrances.

WOODLAND CEDAR BEARD OIL

Makes about ¼ cup

This oil blend is like walking through the forest after a refreshing rain shower. The scent is woodsy, with a lightly sweet floral aroma and a crisp spicy finish. The blend works as a conditioner to moisturize and soften beard hair, and it is wonderful gift to make for yourself or a loved one.

INGREDIENTS

14 drops Virginia cedarwood essential oil

6 drops organic pink pepper essential oil

4 drops organic clary sage essential oil

2 Tablespoons organic jojoba oil

2 Tablespoons organic avocado oil

6 drops vitamin E oil (optional)

DIRECTIONS

1. Drip all the essential oils into a glass bottle.

2. Cap and roll between your palms to combine.

3. Add the jojoba oil, avocado oil, and vitamin E oil to the bottle.

4. Roll between your palms again to combine.

5. Shake before each use.

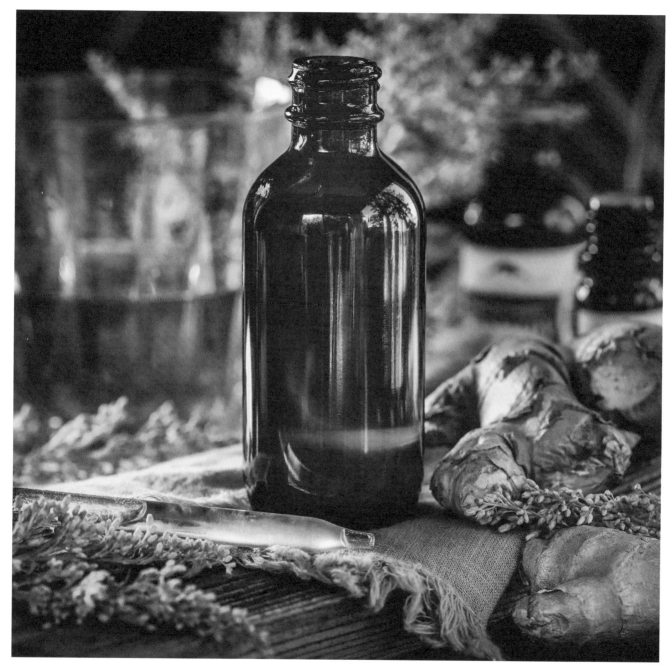

A classic cocktail, the Kentucky Mule, served as the base inspiration for this beard oil.

BOURBON & GINGER BEARD OIL

Makes about ¼ cup

The spicy kick of the ginger balanced against the rich oak and vanilla notes is a drool-worthy combination. Like many great cocktails, this formulation requires a shake before each use because the oakwood absolute tends to separate in oil-based formulations.

INGREDIENTS

10 drops oakwood absolute (see Tips)

1 Tablespoon organic vegetable glycerin

1 Tablespoon organic argan oil

2 Tablespoons organic unrefined almond oil

10 drops organic fresh ginger essential oil

4 drops organic rosemary essential oil

6 drops vitamin E oil (optional)

DIRECTIONS

1. Drip the oakwood absolute into a glass bottle.

2. Add the vegetable glycerin and shake very well to combine.

3. Add the argan oil, almond oil, fresh ginger essential oil, rosemary essential oil, and vitamin E oil to the bottle. Shake to combine.

4. Shake before each use.

TIPS

It can be difficult to measure drops when working with absolutes. Aim for an equal amount of oakwood absolute and fresh ginger essential oil.

To get the absolute to blend well, continue shaking as you add ingredients. The heavenly smell makes the extra effort worth it!

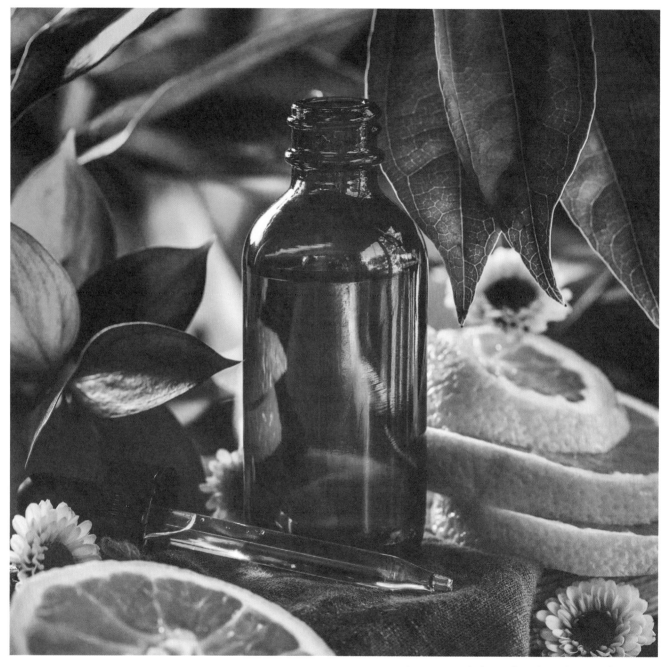

Citrus essential oils in a formulation bring uplifting aroma notes that evoke feelings of clarity and cleanliness.

CITRUS FLOURISH BEARD OIL

Makes about ¼ cup

This gently scented oil blend features uplifting spicy and citrus notes that are balanced by grounding vanilla and balsamic undertones.

DIRECTIONS

1. Drip all the essential oils into a glass bottle.

2. Cap and roll between your palms to combine the essential oils.

3. Add the jojoba oil, pomegranate oil, and vitamin E oil to the bottle.

4. Roll between your palms again to combine.

INGREDIENTS

12 drops elemi essential oil

8 drops organic litsea cubeba essential oil

8 drops amyris essential oil

2 Tablespoons organic jojoba oil

2 Tablespoons organic pomegranate oil

6 drops vitamin E oil (optional)

Radiant
Facial Care

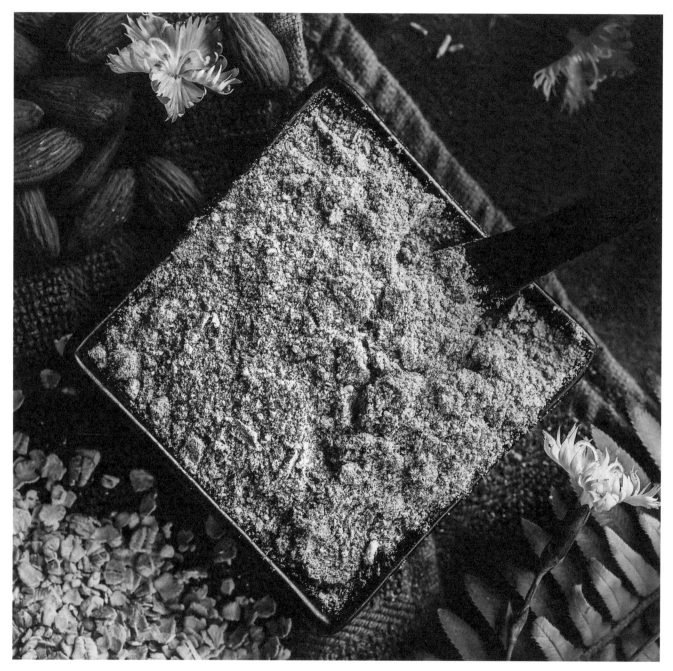

Cleansing grains bring together the cleansing power of clay with natural botanical exfoliants.

GREEN TEA & LAVENDER FACIAL CLEANSING GRAINS

Makes about 3 Tablespoons

Facial scrubs exfoliate the skin and cleanse the pores. Some facial scrubs can be rough on the skin, but this recipe contains oats, almonds, and other nourishing ingredients that are somewhat gentler.

INGREDIENTS

1 Tablespoon organic oats

1 Tablespoon organic almonds

2 teaspoons organic lavender flowers

1 teaspoon French green clay

¼ teaspoon organic matcha tea

2 to 5 drops organic lavender essential oil

DIRECTIONS

1. Grind the oats, almonds, and lavender flowers in a clean coffee grinder until the mixture is a fine powder.

2. Sift through a mesh screen to remove any larger pieces (which may be too abrasive for delicate facial skin).

3. Add the clay, matcha, and lavender essential oil. Mix thoroughly.

4. Store in a glass jar.

TO USE

1. Mix a small amount of the cleansing grains with water, milk, cream, yogurt, hydrosol, or tea to make a smooth paste.

2. Apply to slightly damp skin and gently massage with your fingertips, avoiding the sensitive areas around the eyes and lips.

3. When finished, rinse off with cool water.

TIPS

You can use this same blend for a facial mask. Simply apply a light layer of the hydrated mixture on the face, making sure to avoid the delicate skin area around the eyes and mouth. Leave on for 10 minutes or until the mask feels taut and dry, then rinse off with cool water.

For dry or sensitive skin types, leave the mask on for 5 minutes or less.

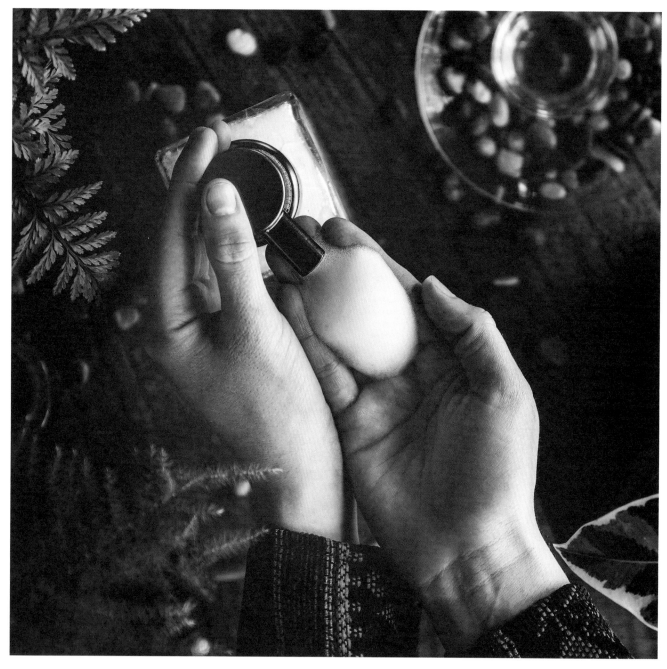

The key to making soap foam is to use a foaming soap dispenser, which you can find at most home goods stores.

FOAMING ROSE FACIAL & HAND WASH

Makes enough for 1 week of daily face and hand washing

When working with recipes that do not contain preservatives, it's important to make them in small batches so they remain free of bacterial growth. This dual-purpose recipe is a great way to go through the recipe quickly, while still enjoying the benefits of preservative-free botanical skin care.

INGREDIENTS

¼ cup organic white rose hydrosol

1 Tablespoon organic castile soap

1 Tablespoon organic rosehip seed oil

1 ½ teaspoons organic pomegranate seed oil

½ teaspoon aloe vera gel

¼ teaspoon vitamin E oil

¼ teaspoon organic vegetable glycerin

2 drops rose absolute (optional)

DIRECTIONS

1. Add all the ingredients to a clean, sterilized bottle with a foam dispensing top.

2. Label with the blend name and date made. Use within 2 weeks.

TO USE

1. Shake the bottle well.

2. Moisten your face with a warm, wet towel.

3. Pump two squirts into your hand and massage the soap into your face for 1 minute.

4. Moisten the towel with warm water and use to remove soap completely.

5. Turn the water to cold and finish by splashing cold water on your face. This will help the pores to shrink back down.

6. Follow up with your favorite moisturizer.

TIPS

Although this recipe contains oil, you'll still want to follow up with a moisturizer.

It's important to use clean sterilized tools and containers to prevent contamination.

This soap also makes a lovely shaving soap!

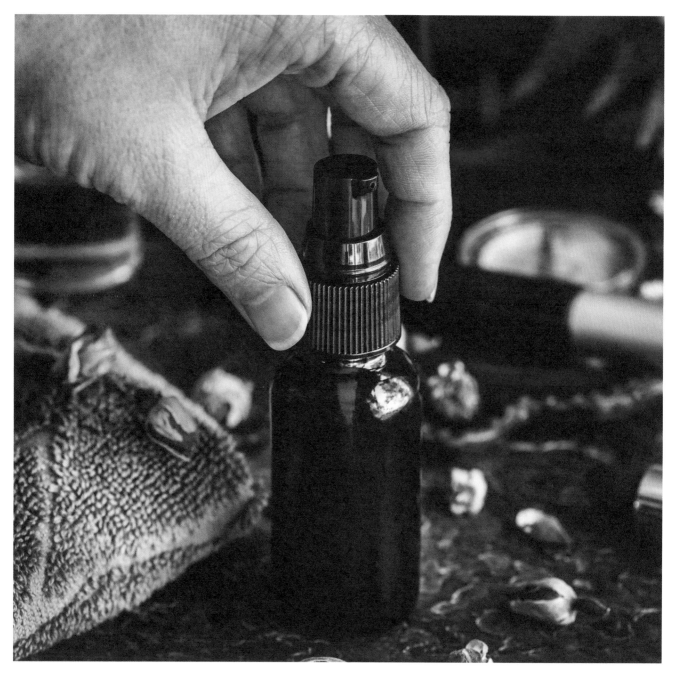

This makeup remover recipe doubles as an excellent facial serum.

HERB-INFUSED MAKEUP REMOVER

Makes about ⅛ cup

This simple recipe is effective, kind to the skin, and easy to customize with herbal allies of your choice. Bonus: use a washcloth or reusable makeup remover pads to save money and say goodbye to single use packaging.

INGREDIENTS

1 Tablespoon herb-infused oil—fennel, rose, or green tea are some of our favorites (prepare ahead)

1 teaspoon organic castor oil

3 drops vitamin E oil

DIRECTIONS

1. Combine all the ingredients in a jar.

2. Cap and shake well to mix.

TO USE

1. Shake the bottle before use.

2. Dampen a reusable facial wipe or cloth makeup remover with warm water and dispense a pea-sized amount of the makeup remover onto the cloth.

3. Gently wipe away your makeup.

4. Rinse the cloth with warm water and wipe down your face again to remove any excess oil or residual makeup.

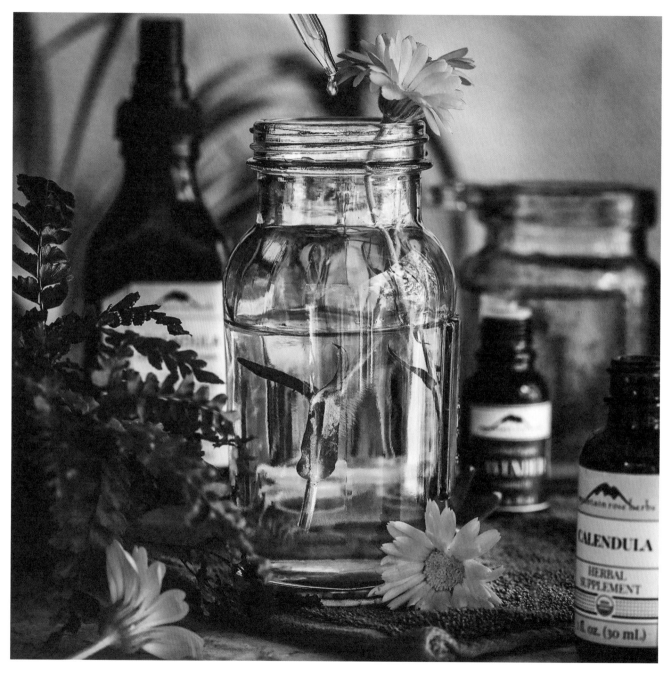

Facial toners help to prime the skin and get it ready to absorb moisturizers and other treatments used after cleansing.

CALMING CALENDULA TONER

Makes about ½ cup

The combination of calendula and lavender makes for a soothing, cooling facial toner. This formulation is wonderful any time of the year, but it comes in particularly handy for hydrating stressed skin in the heat of the day.

INGREDIENTS

½ cup organic calendula hydrosol

15 drops organic lavender essential oil

10 drops organic calendula extract

DIRECTIONS

1. Mix all the ingredients together in a clean glass bottle with an airtight lid. Shake to blend.

2. Pour part of the toner into a 1- or 2-ounce bottle with a mister top. Store the remainder in the refrigerator until ready to use. Refrigerated toner will last up to 1 year.

3. Use as often as desired, shaking to blend before each use.

TIPS

If you are allergic to members of the Asteraceae family (such as feverfew, chamomile, echinacea), consult with a qualified healthcare practitioner before using calendula, as allergic cross-reactivity to Asteraceae plants is common.

Essential oils and extracts can slowly degrade the plastic tube of a spray nozzle over time, so be sure to fill the small mister bottle with only the amount of toner you will use within 2 to 3 weeks. Refill as necessary from the glass bottle that you store in the refrigerator.

This toner is also wonderful for airplane travel when things can get overly warm and uncomfortable. Instead of using a mister bottle, which might disturb your seat neighbors, pour the toner into a 1- or 2-ounce travel-size bottle and bring along some cotton pads. A pad of toner will clean and revitalize your skin on the go.

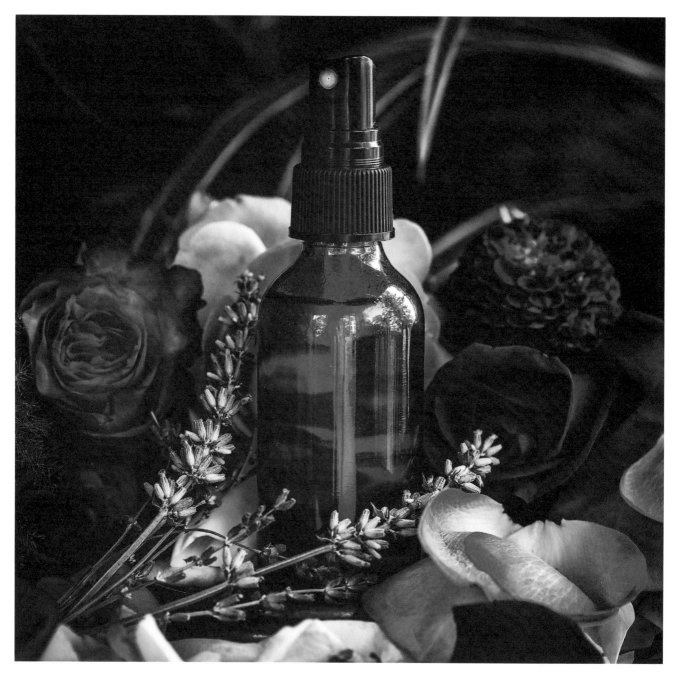

As a humectant, vegetable glycerin helps the skin retain moisture, which is why it works well with light toners and is often a key ingredient in skin care.

ROSE & LAVENDER FACIAL TONER

Makes about ⅜ cup

This gentle toner is perfect for any time of the year. Adjust to your preference—if it feels a little sticky to you, decrease the amount of vegetable glycerin, or if it feels a little drying, increase the vegetable glycerin or add a dash of carrier oil.

DIRECTIONS

1. Place all the ingredients into a clean 6-ounce bottle with a fingertip mister. Shake to blend.

2. This toner should keep for at least 6 months without refrigeration.

TO USE

1. Gently shake before each use as the contents will naturally separate.

2. Wash your face with water, and gently dry it with a soft towel.

3. Mist with the toner and allow your face to air dry or gently pat it dry.

4. Finish by applying a moisturizing lotion, oil, or cream.

INGREDIENTS

¼ cup organic rose hydrosol

⅛ cup organic witch hazel extract

1 Tablespoon aloe vera gel

½ teaspoon organic vegetable glycerin

7 drops organic lavender essential oil

4 drops organic chamomile extract

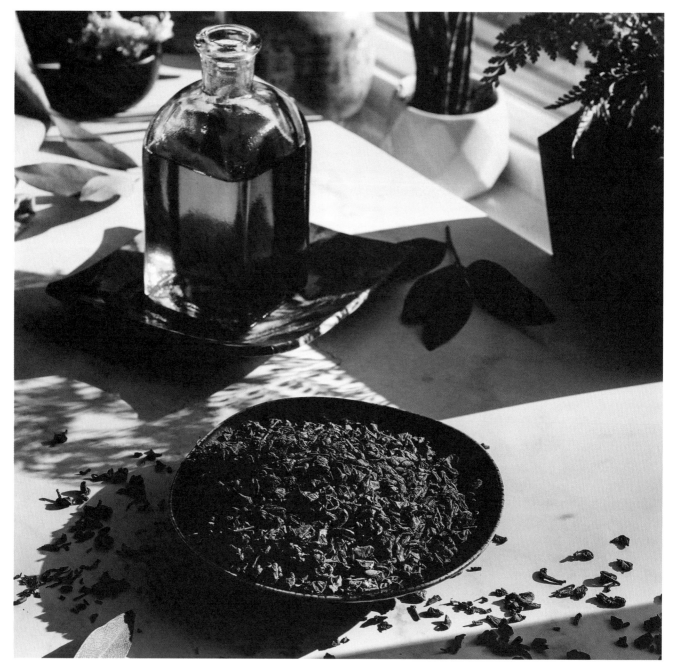

The tannins in green tea help tighten the skin and reduce puffiness.

SKIN FIRMING GREEN TEA FACIAL SERUM

This skin serum calls upon the skin-tightening benefits of tannins, which are found in green tea. Gentle, yet stimulating, this supportive hydrator is suitable for a wide range of skin types and is light enough to use on the face any time of the day.

STEP ONE DIRECTIONS

1. Infuse olive oil with green tea using the herb-infusion method of your choice.

2. When done, strain out the tea leaves and compost or discard them.

3. Pour the strained oil into a storage jar, label with the name and the date made, and store it in a cool, dark place until ready to use.

STEP TWO DIRECTIONS

1. Combine all the ingredients in glass jar with a lid and shake well to combine.

2. Transfer the serum into a dark amber or cobalt blue bottle to protect it from the light and store in a cool, dark place. This serum does not need to be refrigerated and should keep for several months if properly stored.

Step 1: Make Green Tea-Infused Oil

Makes about 1 ½ cups infused oil

1 ⅔ cups organic olive oil

1 cup organic green tea leaves

Step 2: Make Green Tea Skin Serum

Makes about 1 ⅛ cups

½ cup organic green tea–infused olive oil (recipe above)

¼ cup organic avocado oil

¼ cup organic jojoba oil

⅛ cup organic sunflower oil

12 drops organic rosemary essential oil

12 drops organic lavender essential oil

8 drops organic geranium essential oil

4 drops organic myrtle essential oil

TIPS

Any kind of high-quality green tea will work well in this serum.

A little skin serum goes a long way. Use an oil dropper or a low-volume pump to add a small amount of liquid to the palm of your hand, then gently spread the serum over your face with your fingers.

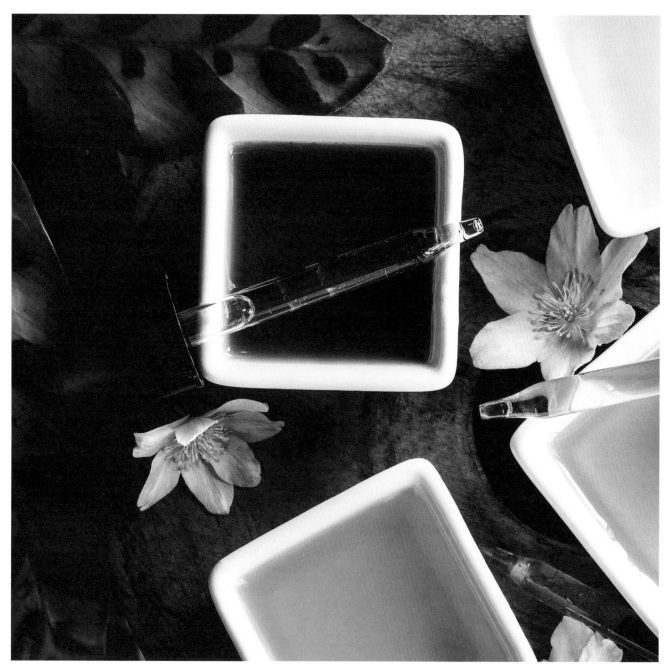

Depending on your skin type, you may use this fast-absorbing serum daily or as a periodic treatment.

NOURISHING SKIN SERUM FOR DRY SKIN

Makes about ½ cup

We have all been fed the beauty myth that oily skin is bad. But what we really need is skin-loving oils like this serum, paired with a nice, gentle astringent for a balanced regimen. Using natural plant oils is a wonderful way to help nourish and refresh dry skin. These oils will absorb into the skin quickly, so they can be used for daily moisturizing.

INGREDIENTS

¼ cup organic jojoba oil or organic sunflower oil

⅛ cup organic tamanu oil

⅛ cup organic rosehip seed oil

1 Tablespoon organic pomegranate seed oil

½ teaspoon vitamin E oil

10 to 20 drops organic lavender essential oil

5 to 10 drops organic carrot seed essential oil

2 to 5 drops organic ylang ylang essential oil (optional)

DIRECTIONS

1. Pour all the carrier oils together into a glass bottle.

2. Cap and roll the bottle between your palms to mix.

3. Carefully drip each essential oil into the bottle and roll again to distribute. Invert the bottle several times and roll again.

TO USE

1. Apply a coin-sized amount as a facial serum and massage into skin.

2. Alternatively, apply small amounts all over your body and massage until absorbed.

TIPS

Use less of the essential oils if you have skin or fragrance sensitivities.

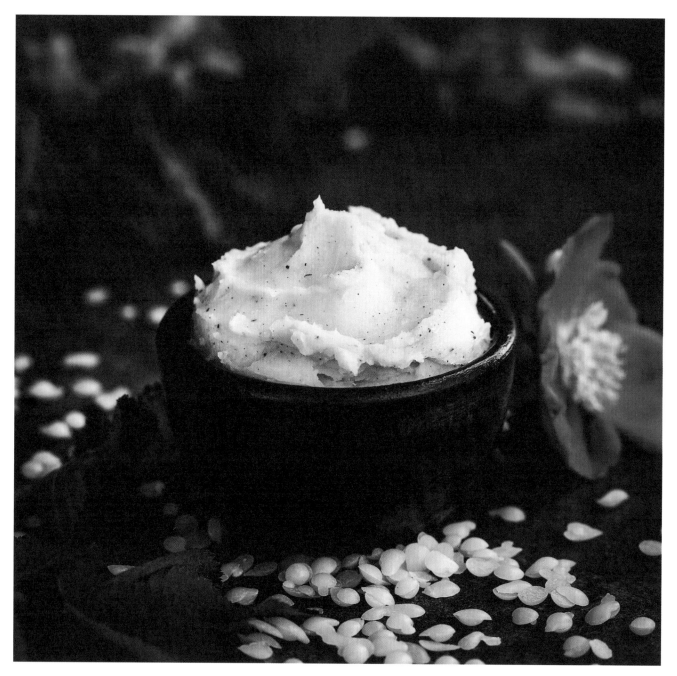

The liquid in a whipped body care recipe must be cold to achieve the ideal consistency.

FACIAL MOISTURIZER
with ROSEHIP SEED OIL

Makes about ⅔ cup

One of the most universally loved oils for facial moisturizers is organic rosehip seed oil. Considered a dry oil—meaning that it is easily and quickly absorbed by the skin without leaving an oily residue behind—rosehip seed oil also contains essential fatty acids that make it beneficial for dry and/or mature skin.

INGREDIENTS

½ cup organic shea butter

2 Tablespoons organic jojoba oil

1 Tablespoon organic rosehip seed oil

⅛ teaspoon organic vanilla bean powder (optional)

1 teaspoon raw local honey

DIRECTIONS

1. Combine the shea butter and jojoba oil in a double boiler over medium heat.

2. Stir until the shea butter melts.

3. Remove the mixture from the heat.

4. Add the rosehip seed oil, vanilla bean powder, and honey.

5. Transfer to a large bowl and stir to combine.

6. Chill the mixture in the refrigerator for 10 minutes or until solid.

7. Use an electric mixer to whip the chilled mixture until fluffy.

8. Transfer to an airtight glass jar.

TIPS

We recommend storing this moisturizer in the refrigerator and using it within 3 months.

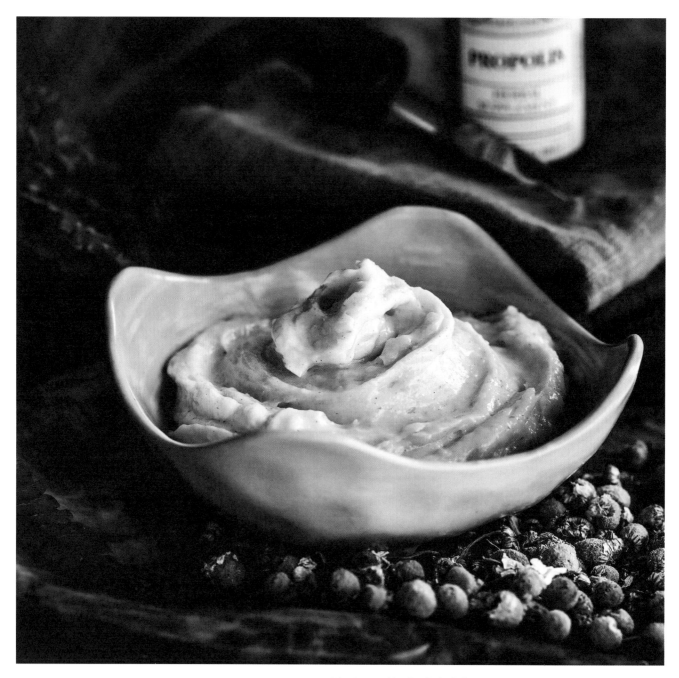

*The skin readily absorbs herbal extracts, but you must add them to hydrating
ingredients to keep them from being overly drying.*

GINSENG & PROPOLIS SKIN EMULSION

Makes about ½ cup

Emulsions are the lightest of the moisturizers. They have fairly thin consistencies and, when infused with botanical extracts, prepare your complexion to face the day without excess oil and shine. The propolis and ginseng in this recipe offer soothing, nourishing support.

INGREDIENTS

¼ cup organic jojoba oil

2 teaspoons beeswax pastilles or grated beeswax

⅛ teaspoon vitamin E oil

¼ cup organic chamomile or calendula hydrosol

¼ teaspoon propolis extract

¼ teaspoon verified forest-grown American ginseng extract

DIRECTIONS

1. Combine the jojoba oil and beeswax in a double boiler over medium heat. Melt the ingredients, while stirring occasionally.

2. Remove from the heat, and stir in the vitamin E oil. Set aside.

3. Pour the hydrosol into a mixing bowl, and add the propolis and ginseng extracts. Blend them together with a hand mixer or emulsion blender.

4. Continue blending constantly as you slowly add the jojoba, beeswax, and vitamin E mixture in small increments. Blend until fully emulsified, when it will have a lotion-like consistency.

5. The finished emulsion can be stored in a salve jar or glass bottle with a treatment pump for 1 to 2 months in the refrigerator.

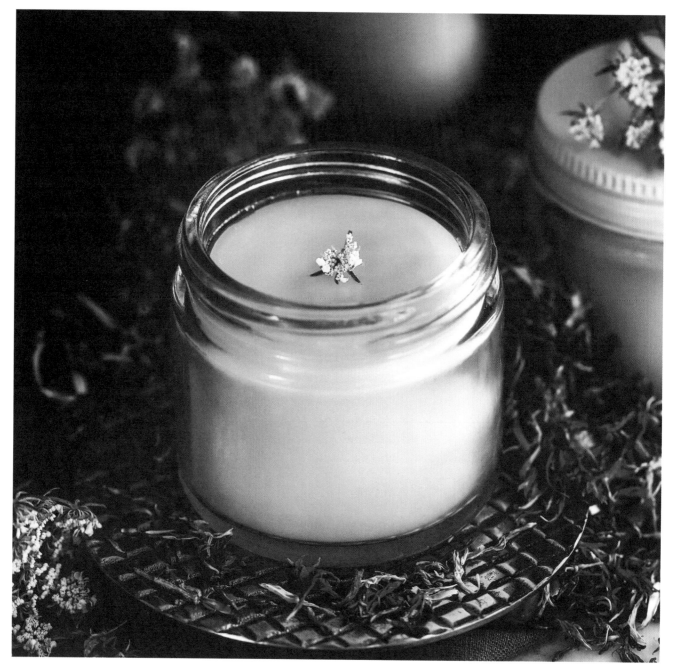

This luscious eye cream is a wonderful addition to evening self-care.

BAOBAB NIGHTTIME UNDER-EYE MOISTURIZER

Makes about ¼ cup

Moisturizing the delicate areas around the eyes helps gently soothe fine lines and wrinkles. Using a gentle touch to apply eye treatments is as important as the treatment itself.

INGREDIENTS

2 Tablespoons organic baobab oil

1 Tablespoon organic unrefined coconut oil (organic refined coconut oil is also okay)

1 Tablespoon beeswax pastilles

1 ½ teaspoons organic refined shea butter

⅛ teaspoon vitamin E oil

DIRECTIONS

1. Place the baobab oil, coconut oil, beeswax, and shea butter in the top of a double boiler over medium heat. Melt the ingredients, while stirring occasionally.

2. Remove from the heat, and stir in the vitamin E oil.

3. Pour the cream into glass jars or tins and let it sit uncovered until the cream solidifies.

4. Cover the containers, and store in the refrigerator.

TO USE

1. After washing your face, gently pat a small amount of the eye cream (less than pea-sized) onto the under-eye area. Be careful to not tug or rub at the delicate skin!

2. Avoid the eyes, waterline, and lashes, and do not apply the cream above your eyes.

3. Gently wash with lukewarm water if cream gets in your eye.

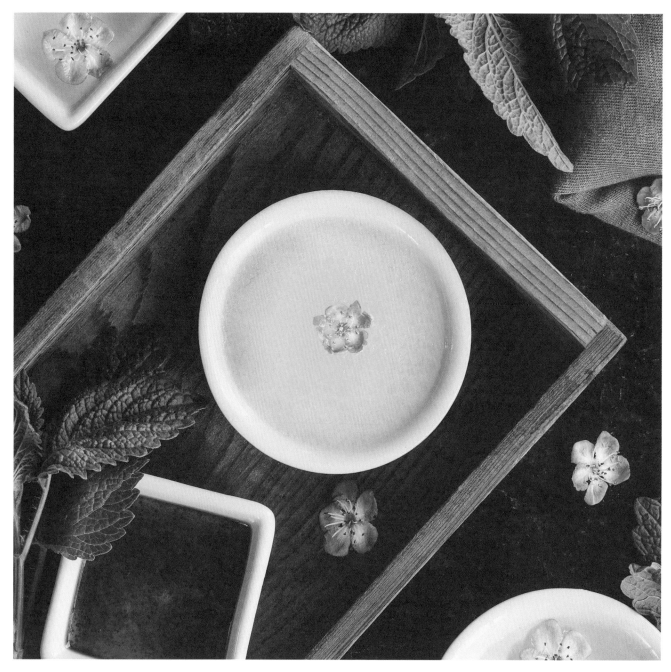

Sheet masks are suitable for all skin types—it's just a matter of mixing the right solution.

HOMEMADE SHEET MASKS

Each recipe makes 1 mask

Sheet masks are an easy and soothing way to relax and pamper at the end of the day. While typically found premade with heaps of preservatives and packaged in single-use plastics and metals, these DIY alternatives offer an economic and sustainable way to consciously care for yourself.

DIRECTIONS

1. Thoroughly whisk together all the ingredients for your preferred mask.

2. Pour the mixture evenly into a wide plate (like a dinner plate).

3. Lay a dry cotton sheet mask over the mixture, and allow the liquid to soak into the fabric.

4. While the mask is soaking, wash your face with a light cleanser.

5. Remove the mask from the mixture and lay it over your face. Position as necessary for proper alignment of the eye and nose holes.

6. Smooth the mask over your skin. Relax for 15 to 20 minutes to let the liquid soak in.

INGREDIENTS

Astringent Sheet Mask for Oily Skin

1 teaspoon organic lemon balm hydrosol

1 teaspoon organic frankincense hydrosol

2 teaspoons organic witch hazel extract

3 drops organic clary sage essential oil (optional)

Hydrating Aloe Sheet Mask for Dry Skin

1 ½ teaspoons aloe gel

1 ½ teaspoons organic calendula hydrosol

½ teaspoon organic pomegranate oil

3 drops organic carrot seed essential oil

Radiant Green Sunrise Sheet Mask for Aging Skin

1 Tablespoon strong-brewed organic green tea

½ teaspoon organic rosehip seed oil

3 drops organic blue chamomile essential oil (optional)

Continued ➔

7. Remove the mask, then gently rub the fabric over your face and neck to help the liquid finish absorbing into your skin.

TIPS

These recipes easily scale up. If you make several fabric masks, you can pre-soak them in a clean container and store them in a refrigerator for up to 2 weeks.

The herbal formulation needs to be thin and liquidy enough to be absorbed by the sheet mask fabric and rinsed out after. Avoid clay masks or other paste-like blends.

You can easily make a reusable sheet mask. (The free Mountain Rose Herbs reusable sheet mask pattern is available here: https://blog.mountainroseherbs.com/little-book-of-body-care-mask-template.) Simply download, print, and cut out to trace onto an absorbent fabric. Cut out the holes and fit slits as directed.

Thin organic cotton jersey works well because it doesn't fray easily when washed, allowing you to use it several times.

Rinse out and air dry your mask after each use to discourage bacterial growth and reduce residue buildup.

Floral Calming Sheet Mask for Any Skin Type

1 ½ teaspoons neroli hydrosol

1 ½ teaspoons helichrysum hydrosol

3 drops organic carrot seed essential oil (optional)

Cucumber Mint Sheet Mask for Sensitive Skin

1 ½ teaspoons organic peppermint tea or organic peppermint hydrosol

1 ½ teaspoons organic cucumber hydrosol

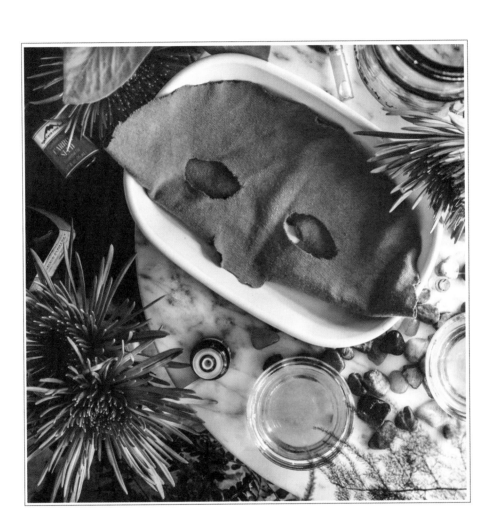

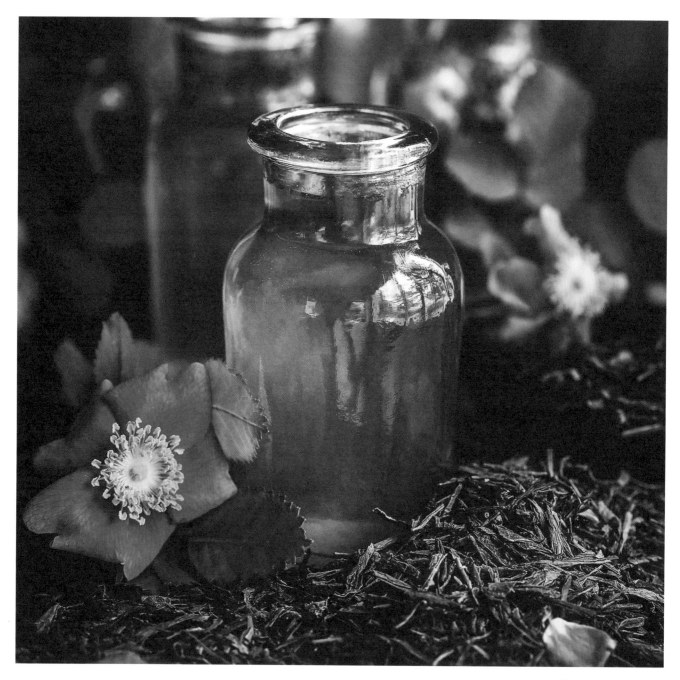

A green tea compress is soothing and encourages you to relax for a few minutes.

GREEN TEA COMPRESS

Makes enough for 1 compress

The difference between a compress and a sheet mask is that compresses are more cleansing and clarifying, while sheet masks are more nourishing. Green tea contains antioxidants that ease and tone the skin and are beneficial for various skin types.

INGREDIENTS

12 ounces of water

2 Tablespoons organic loose-leaf green tea

DIRECTIONS

1. Bring the water to a boil.

2. Pour the boiling water over the tea leaves and allow it to infuse until completely cool.

3. When cool, strain out the leaves and reserve the liquid.

4. Soak a clean cotton cloth in the infusion and place it on your face for 5 to 10 minutes at a time.

5. This process may be repeated several times a day.

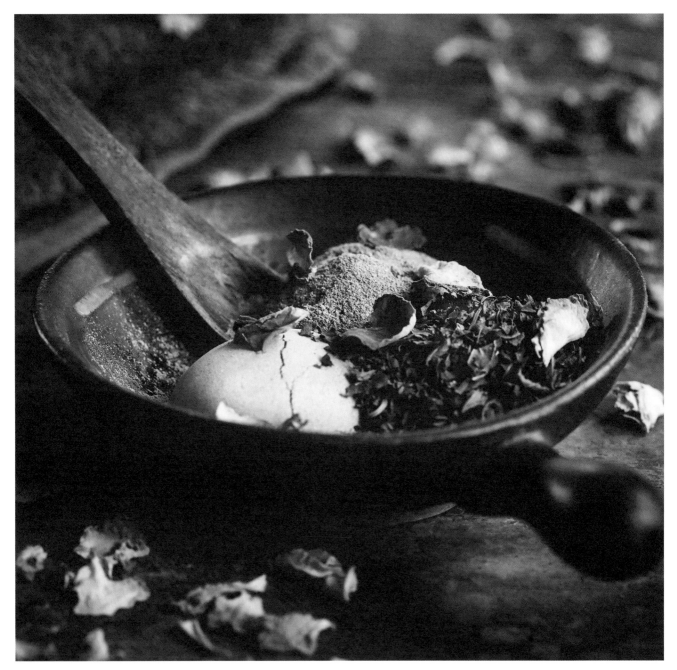

Mixing triphala with neem and peppermint powders creates a simple and effective mask.

AYURVEDIC FACIAL MASK

Makes 1 mask

This recipe is both incredibly easy and quick to take effect. Don't be alarmed if the mixture looks like mud; glamorous skin is revealed after the mask has been removed.

INGREDIENTS

½ teaspoon organic triphala powder

½ teaspoon organic neem leaf powder

½ teaspoon organic peppermint leaf powder (optional)

2 to 3 teaspoons organic rose hydrosol, organic cucumber hydrosol, or organic peppermint hydrosol

DIRECTIONS

1. Mix the powders together in small bowl.

2. Add enough hydrosol to form a soft, muddy paste.

3. Apply the mixture to your face (avoid eyes and areas of sensitivity), and let it sit for 5 minutes.

4. Use lukewarm water to begin removing the mask.

5. Rub your face gently with a washcloth or your bare hands to exfoliate your skin and remove the mask.

6. Rinse your face several times with water to remove the remaining particles.

TIPS

Before using the mixture on your face, try using a bit on your wrist or forearm to see how it feels. If the mixture feels too coarse, omit the peppermint leaf and replace the hydrosols with organic yogurt.

If you feel the need to add moisture back to your face after using the mask, try lightly massaging a few drops of carrier oil into your skin. We like organic almond oil or organic coconut oil. People who have a tendency to get cold skin might prefer a warmer-feeling oil such as organic sesame oil.

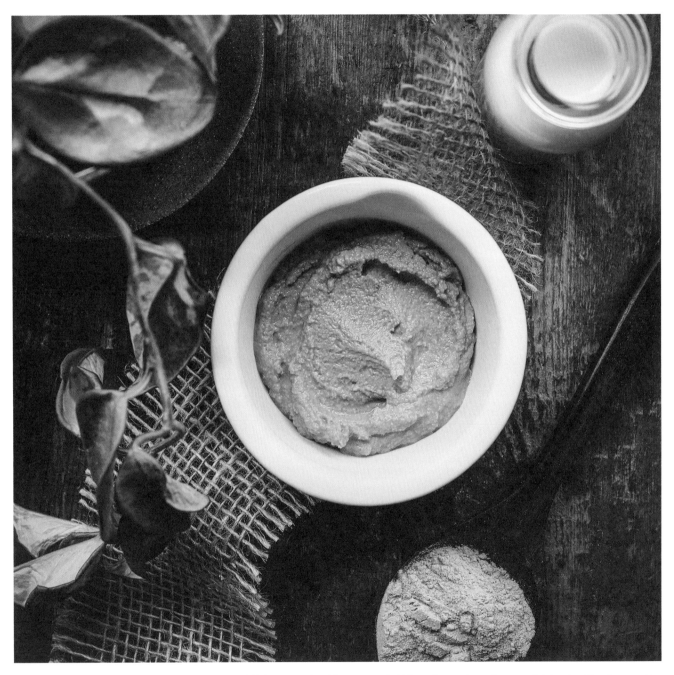

Mixing turmeric with yogurt and chickpea flour reduces the potential that it will stain your skin.

TURMERIC FACE MASK

Makes 1 mask

This simple recipe uses traditional ingredients as well as one unique ingredient: organic turmeric hydrosol. We love how the hydrosol adds a wonderful freshness to the dried powders.

DIRECTIONS

1. Whisk all the ingredients together to form a thick paste; there should be no lumps, and it should feel soft and sticky.

2. Apply the paste to your face with your hands (or a thick brush), and let it dry for 5 to 10 minutes.

3. Wash the paste off with warm water.

4. Pat your face dry with a dark-colored face towel, and rehydrate your skin with a facial toner or facial oil.

INGREDIENTS

2 Tablespoons organic chickpea flour

4 teaspoons organic milk or yogurt (or enough to make a paste)

1 teaspoon organic turmeric hydrosol

1 teaspoon organic turmeric powder

TIPS

We suggest being cautious of other recipes that include turmeric without other dry ingredients.

If you've never used turmeric powder on your skin before, we highly recommend doing a patch test. After Step 1 in the directions above, apply a small amount of the paste to your arm (or somewhere with less sensitivity than your face). Follow Steps 2 to 4, and if you feel that your skin did not react negatively to the paste, you can try the mask on your face.

Continued ➜

Turmeric Face Mask Variations

Turmeric has many healthful applications, and there are a wide variety of turmeric mask recipes used by natural beauty enthusiasts. Honey, oatmeal, and sandalwood powder are a few natural ingredients often used alongside turmeric. A simple web search will give you more ideas, but before you start mixing in your own unique ingredients, it's best to do some research.

If you're worried that turmeric powder will leave a stain on your skin, do a patch test (see above) in addition to decreasing the proportion of turmeric powder used in the recipe. For example, you could start with ¼ teaspoon turmeric powder, and if you are satisfied with the results, you can increase the proportion to a full teaspoon.

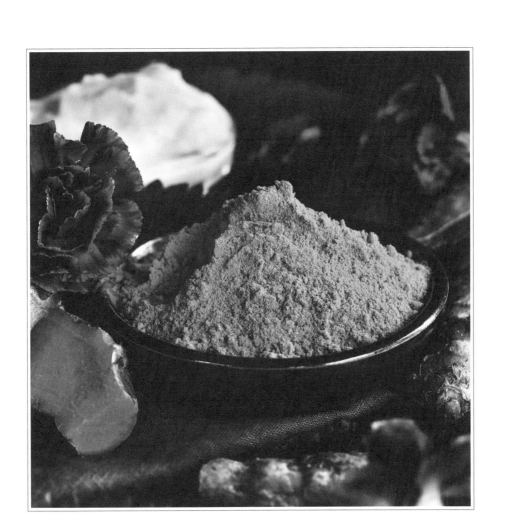

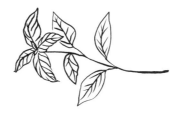

Luscious
Lip Care

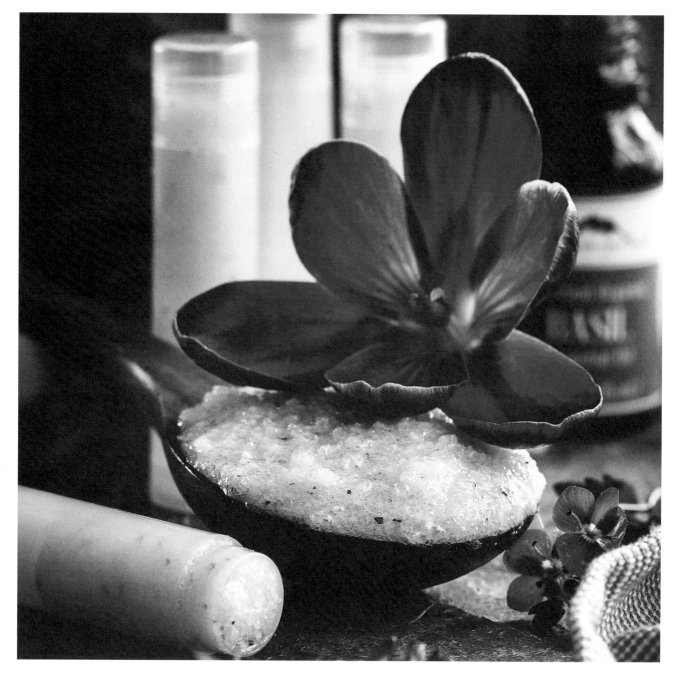

Lip scrubs are an often-forgotten part of lip care.

SWEET BASIL LIP SCRUB

Makes 6 to 8 lip balm tubes

The job of lip balms is to maintain moisture on your lips, but they cannot revive or remove skin that is past the point of no return. That's where lip scrubs come in! This slightly abrasive mixture removes dry layers of skin to reveal the soft, supple tissue beneath.

INGREDIENTS

1 ½ teaspoons organic apricot kernel oil

6 drops organic basil essential oil

1 drop vitamin E oil

2 Tablespoons fine organic sugar

¼ teaspoon organic dried basil leaves

1 ½ teaspoons organic unrefined shea butter

DIRECTIONS

1. Pour the apricot kernel oil, essential oil, and vitamin E oil into a small bowl and stir.

2. Add the remaining ingredients and mix with a fork until it is the consistency of well-combined paste.

3. Pack the mixture tightly into lip balm tubes until full.

TO USE

1. Over the sink or a towel, gently rub the lip balm stick in a circular motion on your lips.

2. Allow the scrub to sit for a few minutes before rinsing off with warm water or wiping it off with a warm washcloth.

3. Pat your lips dry and immediately apply your favorite hydrating lip balm.

TIPS

While this technique sounds like it defies all principles of gravity, we've found that the best way to fill tubes with this scrub is to flip the lip balm tube upside down and press it into the mixture. This technique pushes the scrub into the tube while not making a huge mess.

If you prefer, the scrub can be stored in tins or jars instead. We like the tubes for their ease and tidiness during use.

If you are only making this lip scrub for yourself, you can cut this recipe in half. (You should still share it so you can show off your DIY skills, though!)

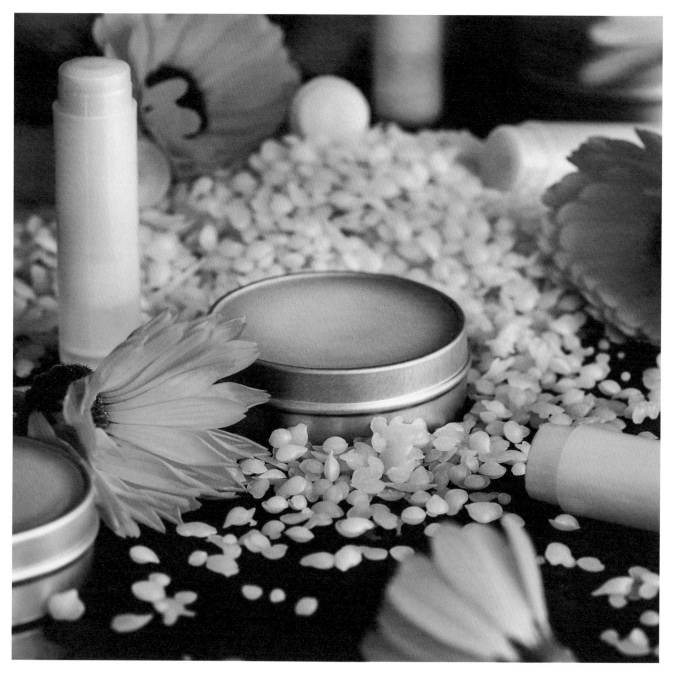

This lip balm recipe also makes a great salve for minor cuts and scrapes.

CLASSIC CALENDULA LIP BALM

Makes about ½ cup

This simple three-ingredient recipe makes a wonderful lip balm or salve. To delight your nose and increase the balm's soothing, balancing properties, we love adding lavender essential oil, but you can change the olfactory profile to make it your own.

INGREDIENTS

½ cup organic calendula herbal oil (or homemade calendula-infused olive oil)

1 Tablespoon beeswax pastilles or grated beeswax

20 drops organic lavender essential oil (optional)

DIRECTIONS

1. Combine the calendula oil and beeswax in a double boiler over medium heat.

2. Heat until the beeswax has melted and is well incorporated with the oil. Remove from the heat.

3. Quickly stir in the lavender essential oil.

4. Pour into lip balm tubes, tins, or glass jars with lids.

5. Allow the balm to cool completely before placing lids on the containers.

6. Store in a cool, dry place. If stored properly, balms can last 2 to 3 years.

TIPS

If your tubes develop air pockets, you can still fix it! Wave a hair dryer around the tube to melt the lip balm and fill the pocket. Be sure to keep the heat source moving so that you don't melt the tube!

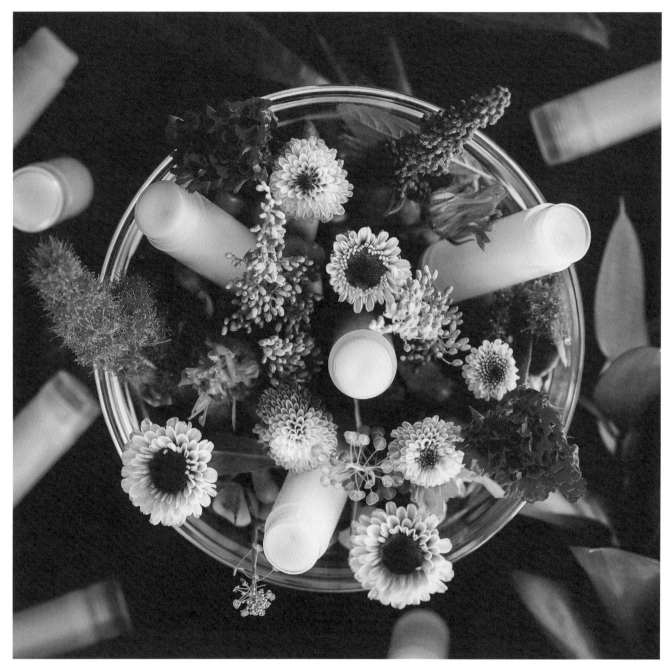

Thanks to their scent and skin-loving benefits, flowers are the most used plant parts in herbal skin care.

FLORAL LIP BALM

Makes 8 to 10 lip balm tubes

Lip balms are easy and satisfying to make, and they are a great self-care tool to always have on hand. This sumptuous recipe is an ode to the lavender-growing regions of the Pacific Northwest. Picture purple-hued fields set against a backdrop of green forested mountains.

INGREDIENTS

1 Tablespoon organic unrefined almond oil

1 Tablespoon organic refined shea butter

1 Tablespoon beeswax pastilles or grated beeswax

8 drops organic lavender essential oil

4 drops cedarwood essential oil

3 drops organic ylang ylang essential oil

DIRECTIONS

1. Gently heat the almond oil, shea butter, and beeswax in the top of a double boiler over medium heat until melted.

2. Remove from the heat, and stir in the essential oils.

3. Pour the mixture into lip balm containers or tins and allow it to cool before placing the lids on.

4. *Optional*: For a polished finish, use a hairdryer or heat gun to smooth the tops after they have hardened.

5. Apply to lips and enjoy!

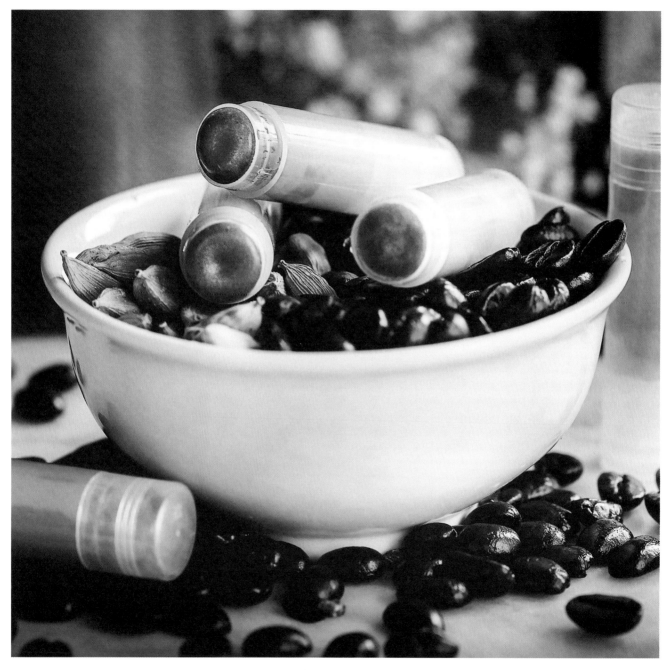

A dreamy pairing of coffee and cardamom makes for a unique and uplifting lip balm.

COFFEE CARDAMOM LIP BALM

Makes 8 to 10 lip balm tubes

This hydrating lip balm evokes the morning wake-up of that first cup of perfect coffee. Put a little pep in your step throughout the day without any coffee jitters.

INGREDIENTS

1 Tablespoon organic unrefined almond oil

1 Tablespoon organic refined shea butter

1 Tablespoon beeswax pastilles or grated beeswax

2 teaspoons finely ground organic coffee beans

14 drops organic benzoin resin essential oil

13 drops coffee absolute

3 drops organic cardamom essential oil

3 drops vitamin E oil

DIRECTIONS

1. Add the almond oil, shea butter, beeswax, and coffee grounds to a double boiler over medium heat.

2. Heat, stirring occasionally, until the oil, butter, and beeswax melt together.

3. Strain through a fine mesh cloth or tea net into a glass or metal container with a spout.

4. Allow the mixture to cool for a couple of minutes.

5. Add the essential oils and vitamin E oil and stir well.

6. Pour the mixture into lip balm tubes, and allow it to cool completely before placing the caps on.

TIPS

Tapping the tube periodically on the counter as you fill it up will help eliminate air bubbles.

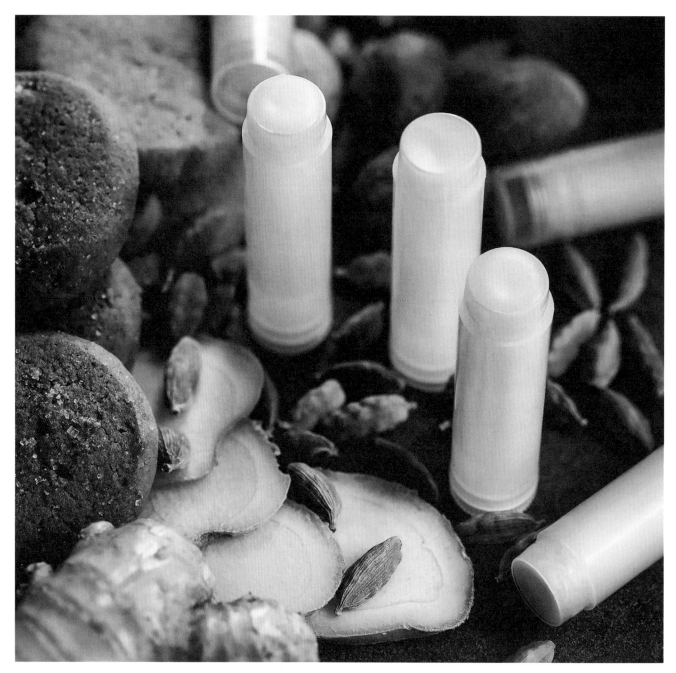

This lip balm was inspired by the winter holidays, but it's wonderful all year round.

ULTRA-HYDRATING GINGER COOKIE LIP BALM

This ultra-hydrating extra-smooth lip balm is bright and uplifting. The natural flavor of marshmallow root imparts a subtle sweetness to lip balm recipes, and the cardamom, fresh ginger, and nutmeg add just the right amount of spice.

INGREDIENTS

2 Tablespoons organic hazelnut oil

1 Tablespoon organic unrefined coconut oil

1 Tablespoon organic roasted cocoa butter

1 Tablespoon beeswax pastilles or grated beeswax

1 Tablespoon organic marshmallow root

6 organic cardamom pods

5 drops organic fresh ginger essential oil

1 drop organic nutmeg essential oil

6 drops vitamin E oil

DIRECTIONS

1. Add the hazelnut oil, coconut oil, cocoa butter, and beeswax to a double boiler over medium heat.

2. When the ingredients are completely melted and incorporated, reduce the heat to the lowest setting and add the marshmallow root and cardamom pods. Infuse for 20 to 25 minutes.

3. Strain the oil using a fine mesh strainer or cotton tea net. Compost the herbs.

4. Add the essential oils and vitamin E oil to the strained mixture. Stir well.

5. Carefully pour the warm mixture into lip balm tubes, tins, or jars.

6. Allow to completely cool before capping.

TIPS

For more aromatic cardamom notes, be sure to break open the pods.

If your lip balm is too soft, remelt it and add more beeswax. If it is too hard, remelt it and add more oil.

Be sure to pour the mixture into the tubes slowly and carefully. Going too fast will cause air pockets to form in the lip balm.

Tapping the tube periodically on the counter as you fill it up will help eliminate air bubbles.

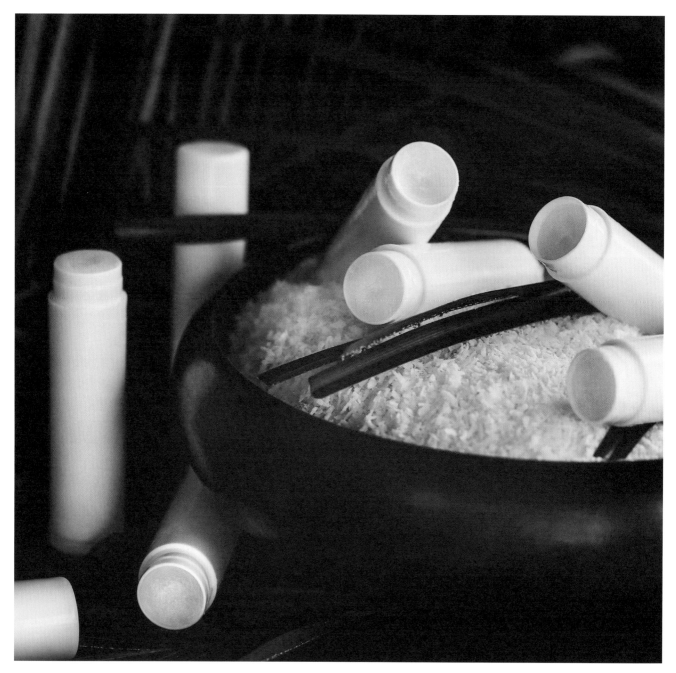

Reminiscent of tropical beaches, this uplifting lip balm blends luscious coconut with notes of ylang ylang and sandalwood.

TROPICAL COCONUT LIP BALM (VEGAN)

People often make vegan lip balms with carnauba wax, which is harder than beeswax. More oil is generally added to these recipes to counterbalance the hardness of the wax. This tropical blend is perfect for warmer weather and for those who prefer a lightweight and glossy lip balm.

INGREDIENTS

2 teaspoons chopped or grated organic carnauba wax

2 Tablespoons organic sunflower oil

1 Tablespoon organic unrefined coconut oil

10 drops organic ylang ylang essential oil

5 drops organic sandalwood essential oil

3 drops vitamin E oil (optional)

DIRECTIONS

1. Place the carnauba wax, sunflower oil, and coconut oil in the top of a double boiler over medium heat, stirring occasionally, until fully melted and incorporated.

2. Remove from heat and stir in the essential oils and vitamin E oil.

3. Immediately pour the mixture into lip balm tubes, tins, or glass jars. Allow it to cool completely before placing caps on the containers.

TIPS

Tapping the tube on the counter periodically as you fill it up will help eliminate air bubbles.

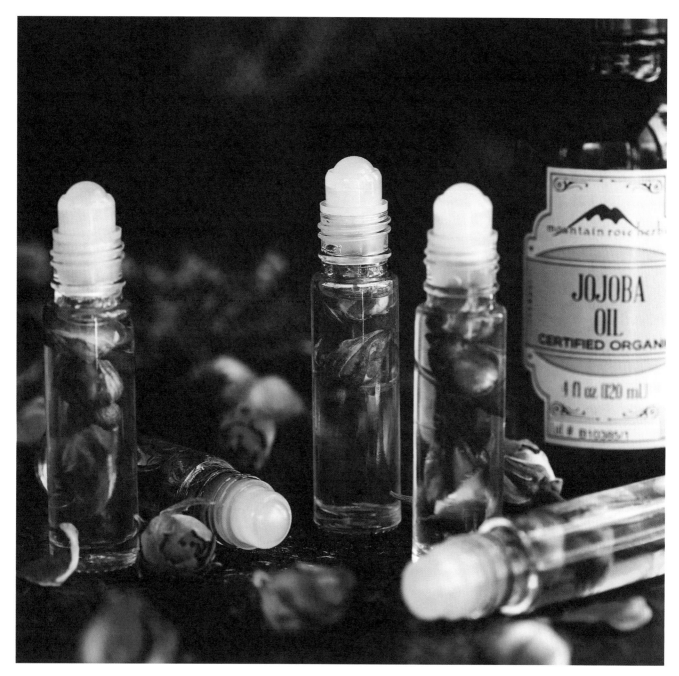

Adding dried herbs and flowers to a roll-top bottle imparts more botanical benefits while adding beauty to your lip gloss.

VEGAN ROLL-ON LIP GLOSS FOR SUMMER

Makes 5 10-ml roll-top bottles

This gloss is the perfect summer solution to keep your lip moisturizer from melting in your pocket, backpack, or on the dash of your car. You'll find the formulation is not as liquified when cold; just put the bottle in your pocket and your body heat will make it perfect again.

DIRECTIONS

1. Combine the jojoba oil and shea butter in a double boiler over medium heat until melted and blended together.

2. Remove from the heat and allow it to cool for 10 to 15 minutes.

3. Stir in the optional vitamin E and essential oil.

4. Place 2 rose buds (or botanical of choice) into each roll-top bottle.

5. Pour the oil mixture into the bottles. Allow it to fully cool before putting on the lid.

6. Shake before use and enjoy!

INGREDIENTS

3 Tablespoons organic jojoba oil

1 Tablespoon organic refined shea butter

2 drops vitamin E oil (optional)

1 or 2 drops organic basil (or other) essential oil (optional)

10 organic rose buds

TIPS

If you choose an essential oil other than basil, you will want to avoid oils that are known to be phototoxic, such as citrus essential oils.

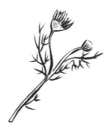

Formulations for Glowing Skin

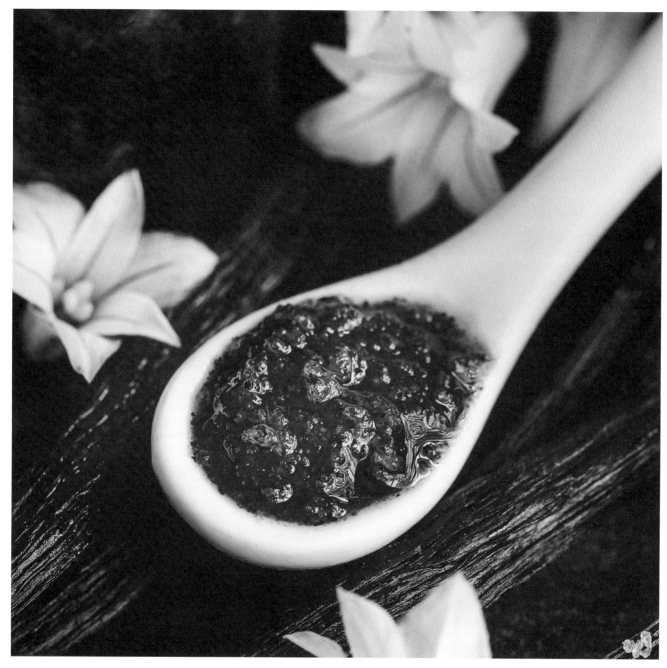

Jojoba meal is created by grinding the seeds after making jojoba oil and makes an exceptional exfoliant.

EXFOLIATING HONEY JOJOBA BODY SCRUB

Honey may be the oldest skin care ingredient known to humans and is particularly nurturing to sensitive skin. The fatty acids found in sweet almond oil, as well as jojoba meal's exfoliating qualities, make this scrub gentler and more moisturizing than some others.

DIRECTIONS

1. In a small bowl, mix together the honey, sweet almond oil, sea salt, jojoba meal, and optional vanilla bean powder until well blended.

2. Add the optional peppermint essential oil and mix well.

3. Take out a bit of the resulting paste and rub it between your hands to check the consistency. The scrub may seem oily in the bowl, but you'll find it absorbs nicely when rubbed into the skin. If it's still too oily, stir in more jojoba meal or fine sea salt.

TO USE

1. Gently massage a palmful of scrub into your wet skin.

2. Rinse off with water.

Makes about ½ cup

INGREDIENTS

½ Tablespoon raw organic honey

3 Tablespoons organic unrefined sweet almond oil

2 to 3 Tablespoons fine sea salt

2 Tablespoons jojoba meal

½ teaspoon organic vanilla bean powder (optional)

1 drop organic peppermint essential oil (optional)

TIPS

If you add too much jojoba meal, the scrub will ball up on your palms like cookie dough instead of spreading evenly with motion. When you thicken the scrub, add more jojoba meal only ¼ teaspoon at a time—just until you reach a grainy paste consistency that easily spreads across the skin.

If you'd like more vanilla scent, you can leave out the peppermint entirely or split a vanilla bean and scrape some of the pulp into the scrub with the vanilla bean powder. Alternatively, you can add a bit of vanilla extract with the peppermint oil.

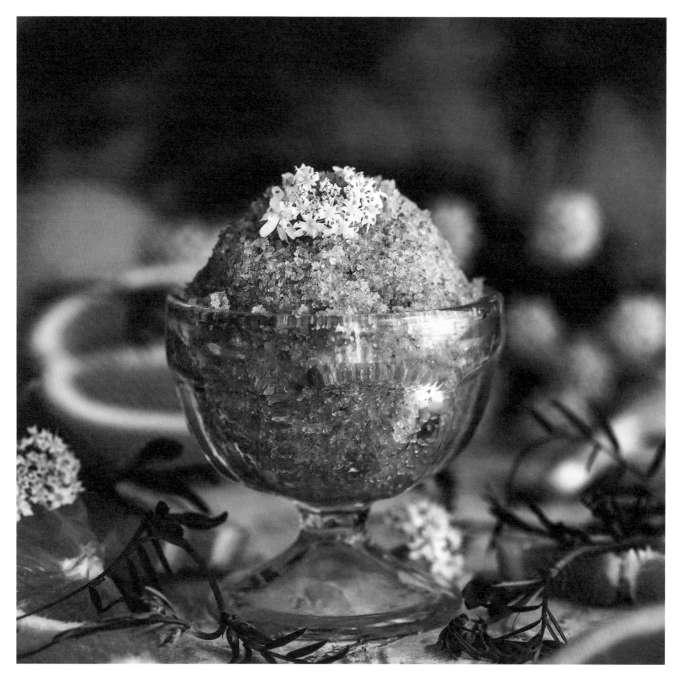

Sometimes the goal of a skin care recipe is to just have fun with the aroma.

ORANGE CREAM BODY SCRUB

Makes about 1 cup

This body scrub was inspired by happy memories of Creamsicles® and summer days. It invites you to embrace the fun and forget about adulting while you scrub away the day.

DIRECTIONS

1. Thoroughly mix all the ingredients in a bowl.

2. Place the scrub in a jar with an airtight lid.

3. Store in a cool, dark, dry place. When stored properly, this scrub will keep for 6 to 8 months.

TO USE

1. Gently massage a palmful of scrub into your wet skin to freshen and exfoliate.

2. Rinse off with water.

INGREDIENTS

¾ cup finely ground Himalayan pink salt or organic raw sugar

¼ cup organic unrefined sweet almond oil

1 Tablespoon liquid castile soap

15 drops organic sweet orange essential oil

5 drops benzoin resin essential oil

TIPS

Oil-based scrubs like this one can make the tub or shower slippery, so use with caution.

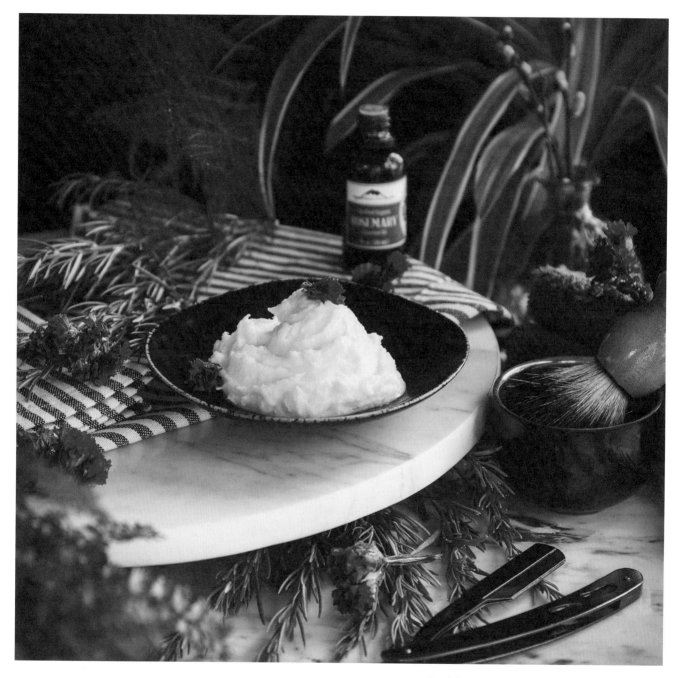

*Good shaving cream uses fats or oils to create a barrier
of friction between the razor and your skin.*

SHAVING CREAM

This fun shaving cream recipe uses only organic ingredients and is fully customizable. Try out different oils, butters, and scents.

INGREDIENTS

4 Tablespoons organic refined shea butter

3 Tablespoons organic unrefined coconut oil

2 Tablespoons kukui nut oil

5 drops organic rosemary essential oil

6 drops organic bergamot mint essential oil

DIRECTIONS

1. Add the shea butter and coconut oil to a double boiler over medium heat. Stir occasionally until the mixture is fully melted and incorporated. Remove from heat.

2. Add the kukui nut oil and essential oils. Stir to combine.

3. Transfer the bowl to the refrigerator and allow the mixture to solidify.

4. Use a hand-held mixer or blender to whip the mixture to a consistency similar to cake frosting.

5. Let the mixture rest for a few minutes, then transfer to an airtight container.

6. This cream will last 1 month if kept away from heat.

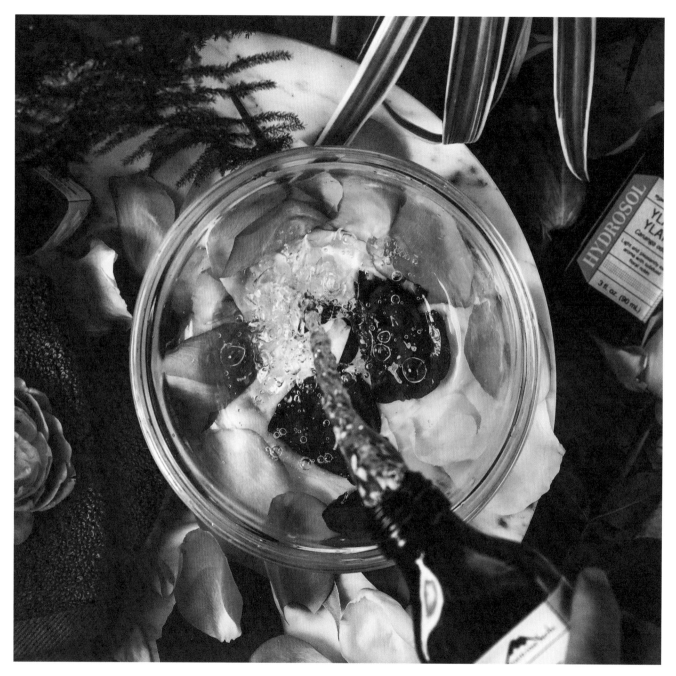

A full body toning mist with glycerin helps skin retain its moisture balance and firmness.

AFTER-SHOWER BODY TONER

Makes about ⅓ cup

Many people use facial toners to help maintain normal pH and hydration of the skin. This after-shower toner pampers the skin from head to toe and can be used daily.

DIRECTIONS

1. Mix all the ingredients in a bottle with a mister top. Put on the mister top and gently shake.

2. Label with the name and date it was made.

3. Store in a cool, dark place. Use within 1 month.

TO USE

1. Shake before each use.

2. Mist your body after a shower or bath.

INGREDIENTS

2 Tablespoons organic ylang ylang hydrosol

1 Tablespoon organic rose hydrosol

1 Tablespoon organic frankincense hydrosol

1 Tablespoon organic vegetable glycerin

¼ teaspoon vitamin E oil

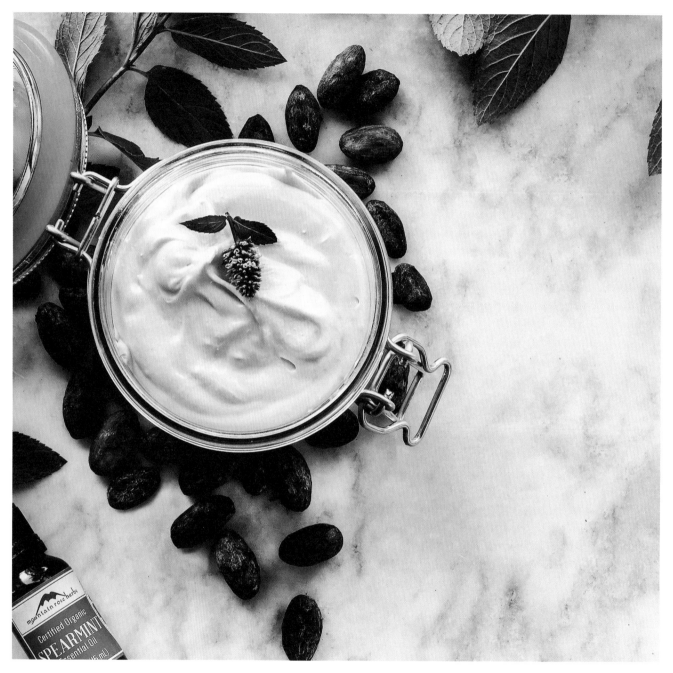

Properly mixing whipped body butters by hand is nearly impossible, but an electric mixer makes it easy.

WHIPPED COCOA MINT BODY BUTTER

Makes about 2 cups

We're all aware of the benefits of drinking plenty of fluids to rehydrate our internal organs, tissues, and cells. But don't forget about the largest organ in your body: your skin. This super-hydrating, cooling body butter is just what your skin needs when it's hot outside or you need an extra dose of moisturizing skin care.

DIRECTIONS

1. Combine the shea butter, cocoa butter, coconut or babassu oil, and rosehip seed oil in a double boiler over medium heat. Gently heat and stir until completely liquefied.

2. Remove from the heat and set aside to allow the mixture to partially cool. You can refrigerate it to speed up this process.

3. When the mixture is just beginning to solidify, whip with an electric hand mixer or stand mixer until the body butter is fluffy. It can help to put the mixing bowl into an ice bath as you blend.

4. Whip in the vitamin E oil and spearmint essential oil.

5. Add the cocoa absolute, and whip again until stiff peaks form.

6. Spoon the body butter into jars or tins.

INGREDIENTS

½ cup organic refined shea butter

½ cup organic roasted cocoa butter

½ cup organic unrefined coconut oil or organic babassu oil

½ cup organic rosehip seed oil

2 teaspoons vitamin E oil

¾ teaspoon organic spearmint essential oil

¾ teaspoon cocoa absolute

TIPS

Adding the cocoa absolute at the end, by itself, helps it to incorporate more thoroughly. You'll want to whip until you don't see any streaks of absolute in the creamy butter.

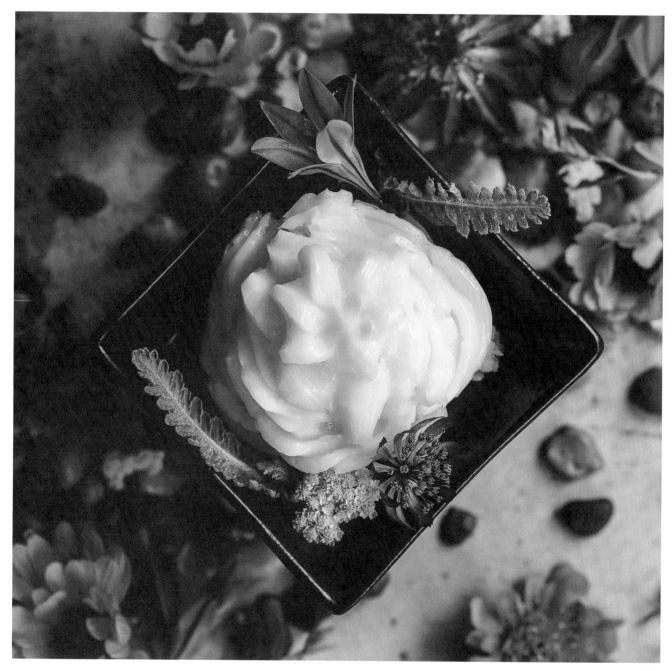

Consider sustainability and choose only reputable suppliers
when purchasing sandalwood essential oil.

LUSCIOUS WHIPPED SANDALWOOD BODY BUTTER

Makes about 1 cup

There is something so luxurious about a fluffy, buttery, moisturizing body butter scented with sandalwood. If you're looking for a super-moisturizing recipe, this one is a good choice.

DIRECTIONS

1. Place the shea nut oil, mango butter, and pomegranate seed oil into the top of a double boiler over medium heat. Heat on medium and stir until the ingredients are fully melted together, leaving no chunks of butter behind.

2. Once melted, turn off the heat and stir in the sandalwood essential oil and vitamin E oil.

3. Place in the refrigerator for 20 to 40 minutes, until the mixture starts to thicken.

4. Using a handheld mixer, whip the thickened oils and butters until it reaches a fluffy consistency. (If you tried this too soon in the cooling and thickening process and the mixture doesn't fluff up as desired, just put it back in the refrigerator.)

5. Once fluffy, scoop the whipped butter into containers. You can also put it in a pastry bag or a plastic bag with a clipped corner and squeeze it into your container(s) of choice.

INGREDIENTS

½ cup shea nut oil

½ cup mango butter

2 Tablespoons organic pomegranate seed oil

50 drops organic sandalwood essential oil

1 teaspoon vitamin E oil

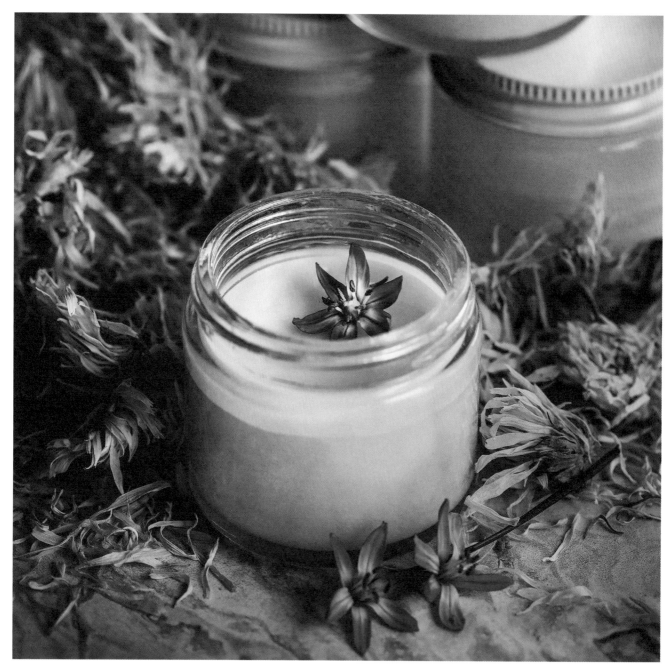

Homemade belly butter made with nourishing ingredients relieves discomfort and redness and helps the skin maintain its elasticity during and after pregnancy.

MAMA'S BELLY BUTTER

Makes about 1 ⅓ cups

To those of you who are pregnant or planning to have a child, congratulations! May this easy-to-make belly butter bring you soothing care and support on your journey. This recipe also makes a wonderful gift for friends and family who are expecting.

INGREDIENTS

½ cup organic roasted cocoa butter wafers

¼ cup organic babassu or coconut oil

¼ cup organic calendula herbal oil (or homemade calendula-infused olive oil)

2 Tablespoons organic shea butter

1 Tablespoon organic rosehip seed oil

2 Tablespoons beeswax pastilles or grated beeswax

Up to 15 drops vitamin E oil

Up to 50 drops organic lavender essential oil (optional)

DIRECTIONS

1. In a double boiler over medium heat, gently warm the cocoa butter, babassu or coconut oil, calendula oil, shea butter, rosehip seed oil, and beeswax just until melted, stirring occasionally to incorporate.

2. Remove from heat.

3. Stir in the vitamin E oil and optional lavender essential oil.

4. Pour into tins or jars. Allow to cool before putting on lids.

TO USE

1. For maximum hydration, rub the butter onto your belly in a soothing motion twice a day.

2. Remember that the rest of you is also working hard to accommodate and carry your child. Your hips, thighs, breasts, and shoulders will also appreciate some soothing balm.

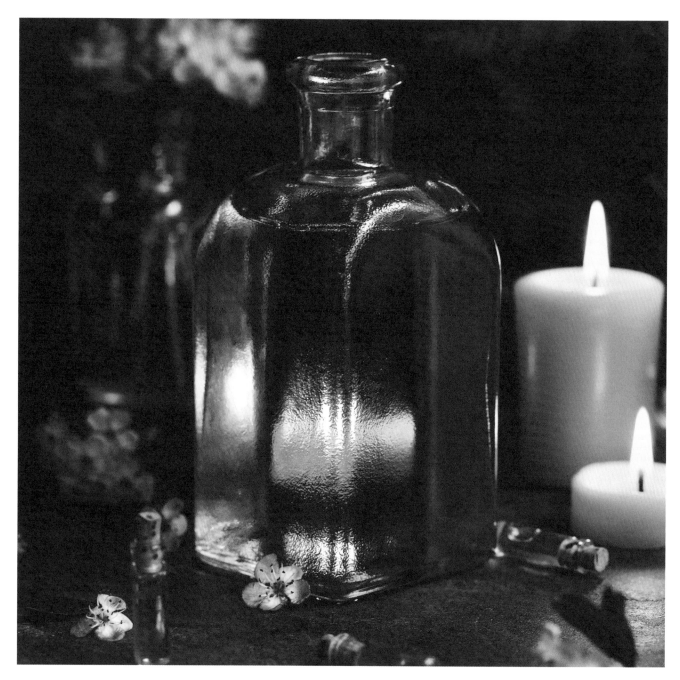

Massage oils are one of the easiest DIY preparations to craft.

MASSAGE OIL

Makes about 1 cup

Massage offers a host of health benefits. It relieves tight or sore muscles, helps improve blood flow and circulation, and is a great way to ease an overactive mind. Skin-loving massage oils are simple to make and customize to match your personal goals. Some of the best organic carrier oils to use for massage oil are:

> Herb-infused oils of your choice
> Calendula herbal oil
> Fractionated coconut oil
> Jojoba oil
> Olive oil
> Rosemary herbal oil
> Sunflower oil
> Sweet almond oil

A range of aromatherapeutic essential oils can be used in this recipe.
Top notes Bergamot, grapefruit, mandarin, peppermint, sweet orange
Middle notes Cardamom, chamomile, clary sage, fir needle, geranium, lavender, neroli, petitgrain, ylang ylang
Base notes Cedarwood, frankincense, patchouli, sandalwood, vanilla, vetiver

INGREDIENTS

65 to 90 drops essential oil(s)

1 cup organic carrier oil

½ teaspoon vitamin E oil

Continued →

DIRECTIONS

1. Drip the essential oils into a plastic or glass bottle with a pump top or one that is easily pourable.

2. Add the carrier oil of your choice and the vitamin E oil.

3. Secure the lid and roll the bottle between your palms to blend the oils.

4. Before each use, roll the bottle between your palms to reblend the oils.

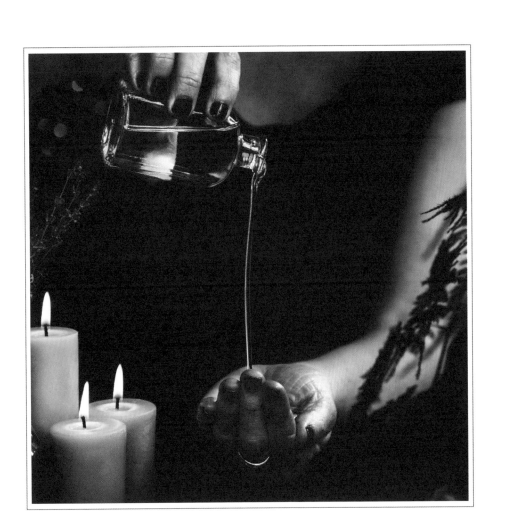

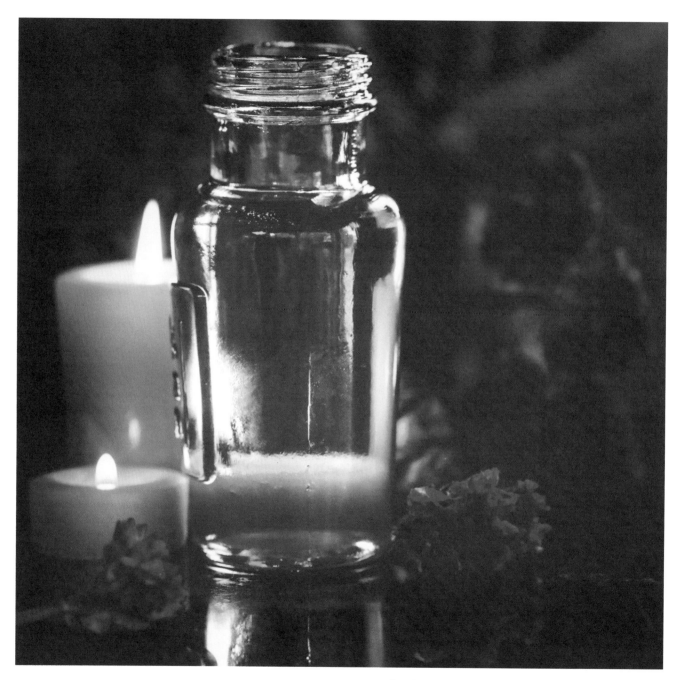

The relaxing energetics of hemp helps to promote restful slumber.

DREAMY HEMP BLEND MASSAGE OIL FOR SLEEP

Makes about 1 cup

Use this massage oil for self-massage or with a partner before bed for muscle relaxation and to support a good night's sleep. Hemp essential oil does not contain traceable quantities of tetrahydrocannabinol (THC) or cannabidiol (CBD). Its use in this recipe is for its dreamy aromatherapy properties.

INGREDIENTS

¼ teaspoon organic hemp essential oil

½ teaspoon organic benzoin resin oil

24 drops organic bergamot essential oil

8 drops organic blue chamomile essential oil

1 cup kukui nut oil

½ teaspoon vitamin E oil

DIRECTIONS

1. Drip the essential oils into a bottle with a pump top or one that is easily pourable.

2. Add the kukui nut oil and vitamin E oil.

3. Securely put on the pump top and roll the bottle between your palms to blend.

4. Before each use, roll the bottle between your palms to reblend the oils.

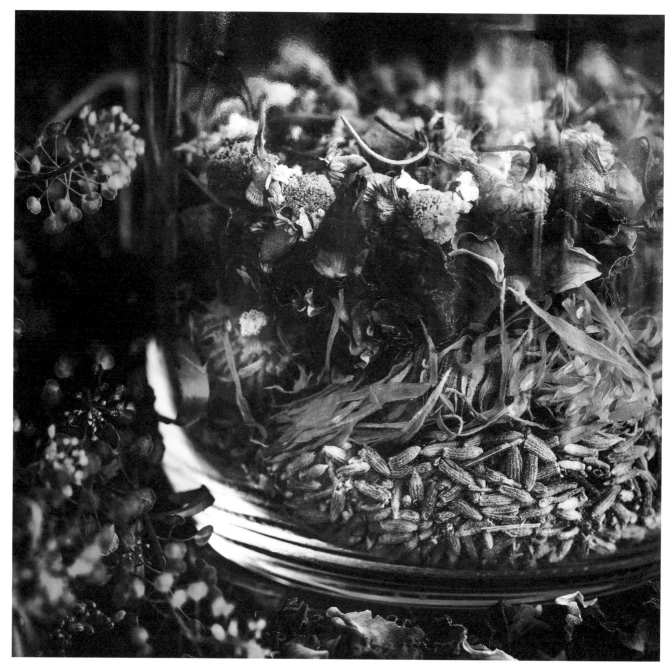

When creating recipes for breastfeeding moms and babies, every ingredient must be safe for infants.

FLOWER-INFUSED OIL FOR BABY & MOM MASSAGE

Makes about 2 cups

This soothing and gentle massage oil is perfect for nurturing baby's sensitive skin. Massage into skin after bath time to reduce dryness, stimulate healthful circulation, and activate developing muscles. This oil blend is also good for helping to rejuvenate postpartum skin and give tired mom muscles some much needed stress relief.

DIRECTIONS

1. Infuse carrier oil of choice with the rose petals/buds and chamomile, lavender, and calendula flowers (prepare ahead).

2. Strain and then stir in the vitamin E oil.

3. Pour into an air-tight glass bottle.

4. Store in a cool, dark place. Depending on the shelf life of the oil used, this blend will be shelf stable for 6 months to a year.

INGREDIENTS

1 ¼ cups gentle carrier oil(s) of choice (favorites for baby include organic sunflower oil, sesame oil, sweet almond oil, and fractionated coconut oil)

¼ cup organic lavender flowers

¼ cup organic calendula flowers

2 Tablespoons organic rose petals or buds

2 Tablespoons organic chamomile flowers

½ teaspoon vitamin E oil

TIPS

Pour a small amount of the flower-infused oil into bathwater for a luxurious pampering soak, but be mindful when exiting as the tub can become slippery.

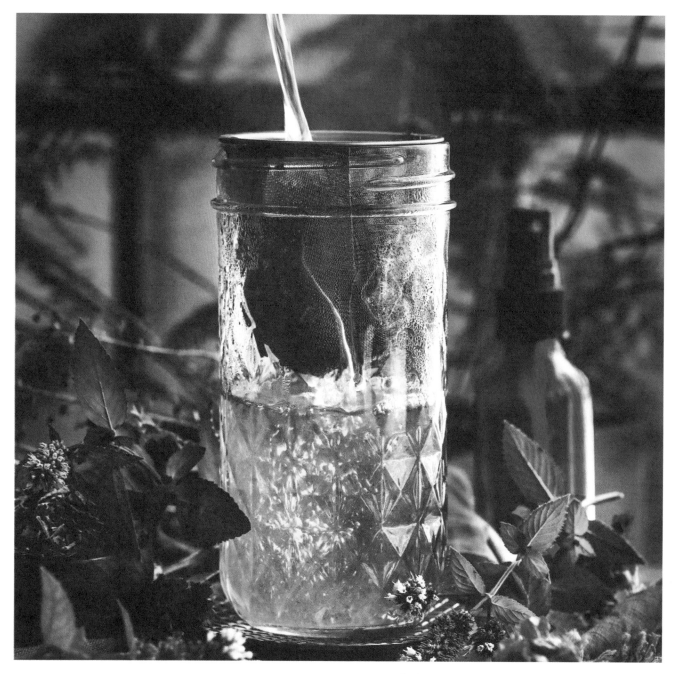

Refreshing peppermint and soothing green tea create the perfect body and face spray when you need to cool off.

PEPPERMINT & GREEN TEA COOLING MIST

Makes about ¾ cup

Use this mist whenever you're in need of a little cooling off. Peppermint is very refreshing, and the green tea in the blend helps reduce redness.

¾ cup distilled or purified water

2 Tablespoons organic peppermint leaf

1 teaspoon organic green sencha leaf tea

1 to 2 drops organic peppermint essential oil (optional)

DIRECTIONS

1. Bring the water to a boil, then pour it over the peppermint and green sencha tea leaves. Cover and infuse until cool.

2. Strain out the leaves and pour the liquid into a 4-ounce spray bottle.

3. Add the optional essential oil, cap the bottle, and shake to combine.

4. Use within 1 to 2 days or store in the refrigerator for up to a week.

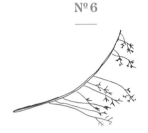

Support for Hard-Working Hands & Feet

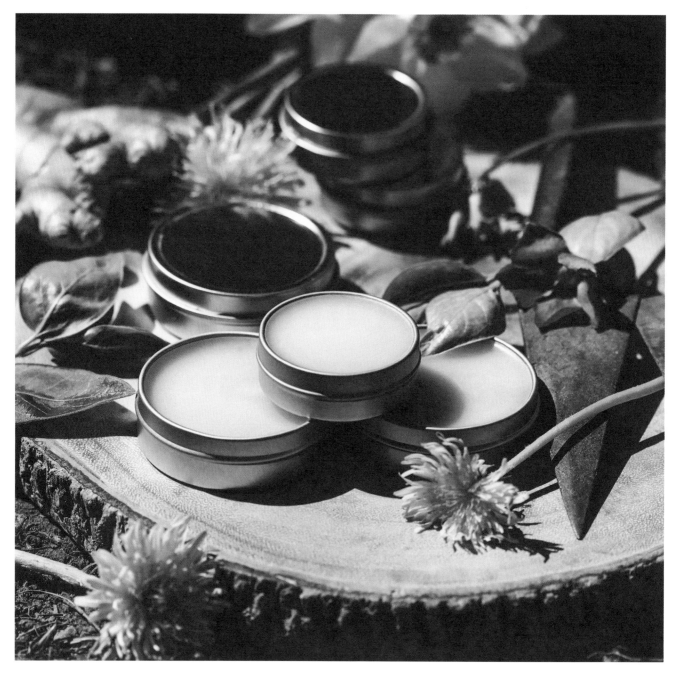

This salve features herbs and oils that bring comfort and support to roughened, tired skin.

SOOTHING GARDENER'S SALVE

Makes about 1 ¼ cups

We love getting our hands in the dirt, and this salve is perfect to use after an afternoon working in the garden. It's also a good recipe to experiment with: make half a batch with herb-infused oil and the other half with plain olive oil to see the difference that a botanical infusion makes.

DIRECTIONS

1. Combine arnica oil, ginger oil, and beeswax in a double boiler over medium heat. Heat just until the beeswax has melted and the mixture is incorporated.

2. Stir quickly to combine, then remove from the heat.

3. Working quickly so the beeswax does not start to solidify again, thoroughly stir in the rosehip seed oil, vitamin E oil, and essential oils.

4. Pour the mixture into storage tins. Allow the salve to cool completely before putting on the lids.

5. Store in a cool, dry place. If stored properly, salves can last for 2 to 3 years. However, if you're a hands-on gardener, these tins aren't likely to be around for too long!

INGREDIENTS

½ cup organic arnica-infused olive oil

½ cup organic ginger-infused olive oil

¼ cup beeswax pastilles or grated beeswax

1 Tablespoon organic rosehip seed oil

1 Tablespoon vitamin E oil

20 drops organic lavender essential oil

20 drops organic ginger essential oil

TIPS

If you opt for DIY arnica- and ginger-infused oils, we've found that filling a 7-ounce pantry jar three-quarters full with organic arnica flowers and another 7-ounce pantry jar half full with the organic dried ginger root, then topping off with oil, was a good amount of herb for this recipe.

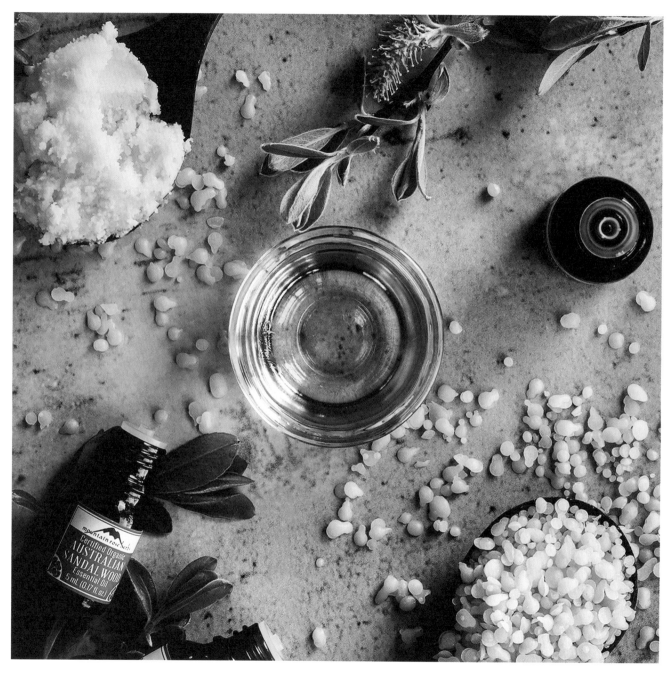

Keeping your cuticles well hydrated is the key to avoiding splitting or breaking, which can leave your nail beds vulnerable to infection and injury.

ARGAN OIL CUTICLE CREAM

Makes about ½ cup

Cuticles get a little unruly at times if not properly cared for, but they serve an important purpose. Their job is to protect our nail beds, so it behooves us to protect them. Maintaining well-hydrated cuticles is what keeps them strong and manageable.

INGREDIENTS

2 Tablespoons organic argan oil

2 Tablespoons organic unrefined sweet almond oil

1 Tablespoon + 1 teaspoon beeswax pastilles or grated beeswax

2 Tablespoons organic unrefined shea butter

3 drops vitamin E oil

20 drops organic Australian sandalwood essential oil or organic lavender essential oil

10 drops organic sweet orange essential oil

10 drops organic tea tree essential oil

DIRECTIONS

1. Add the argan oil, sweet almond oil, beeswax, and shea butter to the top of a double boiler over medium heat. Gently heat, stirring occasionally, until fully melted together.

2. Remove from the heat and thoroughly stir in the vitamin E oil and essential oils.

3. Quickly pour the mixture into tins or jars. Let the mixture cool before placing the lids on the containers.

TO USE

1. Soak your nails in warm, soapy water for at least 5 minutes, then pat dry.

2. Gently push your cuticles back with something soft, such as a cuticle stick made of wood or firm rubber.

3. Rub the nourishing cream into your cuticles

TIPS

Keep a tin of this cuticle cream wherever you're likely to use it regularly—in your bathroom, on your nightstand, or even at your work desk. With regular use, you'll find that your cuticles are less irritated, with the added benefit of fewer hangnails and an overall improvement in nail appearance and resilience.

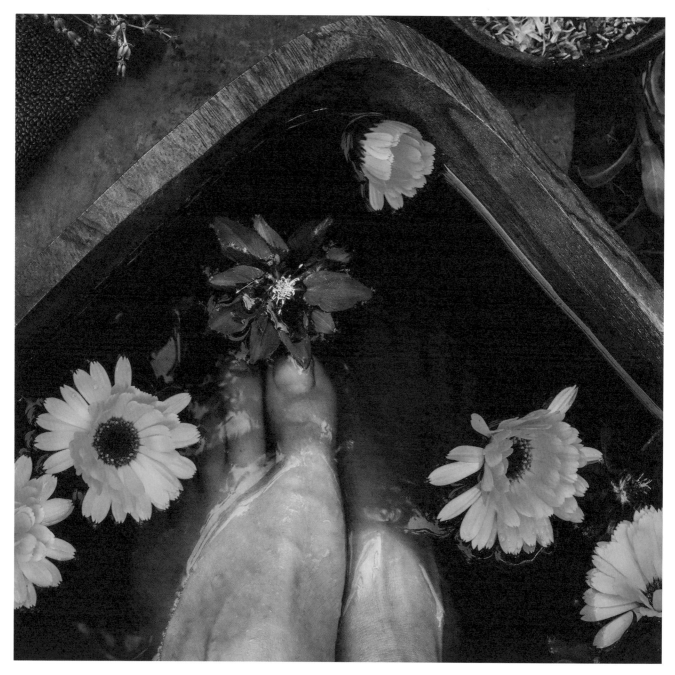

*Treating yourself to a warm herbal foot soak after a long
day releases tension and is deeply cleansing.*

FOOT SOAK
with HERBS

We like to make big batches of this herb mixture and store the excess in a large pantry jar. Feel free to experiment with different ratios and herbs. Some of the best herbs for foot soaks include:

- › Chamomile flowers
- › Holy basil leaf
- › Lemon balm leaf
- › Oat tops
- › Peppermint leaf
- › Red clover blossoms
- › Rose petals
- › Rosemary leaf

INGREDIENTS

1 cup organic calendula flowers

1 cup organic lavandin or lavender flowers

2 cups organic comfrey leaf (optional)

Epsom salt (optional)

TIPS

Comfrey should only be used topically on healthy, unbroken skin. If necessary, substitute with one of the other herbs listed above.

After a foot bath is the perfect time to exfoliate and moisturize your feet.

DIRECTIONS

1. Combine the herbs together in large bowl and stir until thoroughly mixed.

2. Fill a large drawstring muslin bag with the herbs and tie it closed.

3. Place the bag in a foot soak basin and pour hot water (approximately 1 gallon) over it. Let it steep to create a tea.

4. Add a few tablespoons of Epsom salt, if desired.

5. Once the water is at a comfortable temperature, place your feet in the basin, sit back, and enjoy!

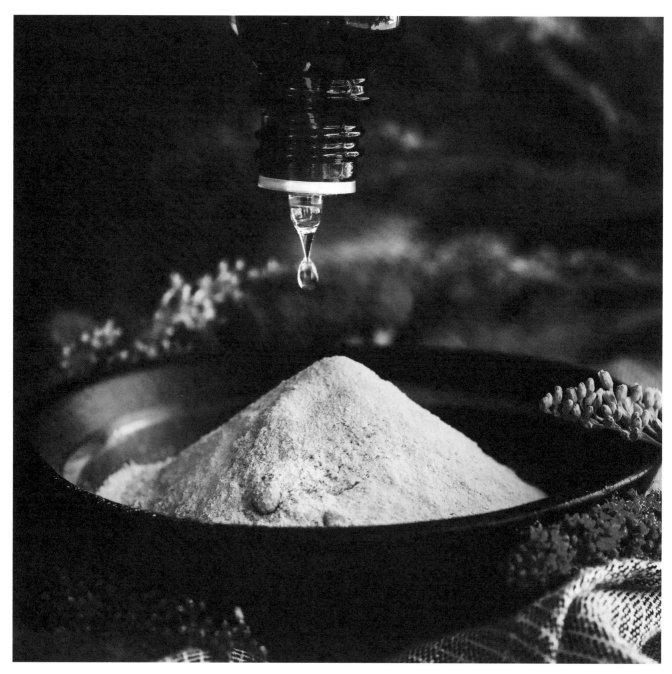

Clay foot masks go deep to remove impurities while also softening the skin.

FOOT MASK

Makes about ⅓ cup

Like other masks, a foot mask helps to sluff off old skin, smooth, moisturize, and boost circulation. Applying a foot mask is also a great excuse to sit down and take a little time for yourself.

INGREDIENTS

3 Tablespoons bentonite clay

3 to 4 Tablespoons raw organic apple cider vinegar

5 drops organic tea tree essential oil

DIRECTIONS

1. Find a place where you can sit comfortably with your feet up for 15 to 30 minutes.

2. Prepare a basin with warm water, and place towels and a pair of socks near where you'll be sitting.

3. Measure the clay in a glass or ceramic bowl.

4. Add the apple cider vinegar one tablespoon at a time and mix until you achieve a paste that is the desired consistency.

5. Add the tea tree essential oil and mix well.

6. Apply a thin layer to the entire foot including between your toes. Leave on for 15 to 30 minutes.

7. Soak your feet in the wash basin and use a washcloth to help remove the clay. If needed, complete the rinse-off in a shower. Always be mindful when walking after foot treatments, as your feet may be slippery!

8. Fully dry your feet, and put on socks to keep your feet clean and prevent slipping.

TIPS

Because a large amount of clay can clog drains, we recommend dumping the foot basin outside when you're finished.

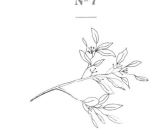

7

Shower & Bath Enhancements

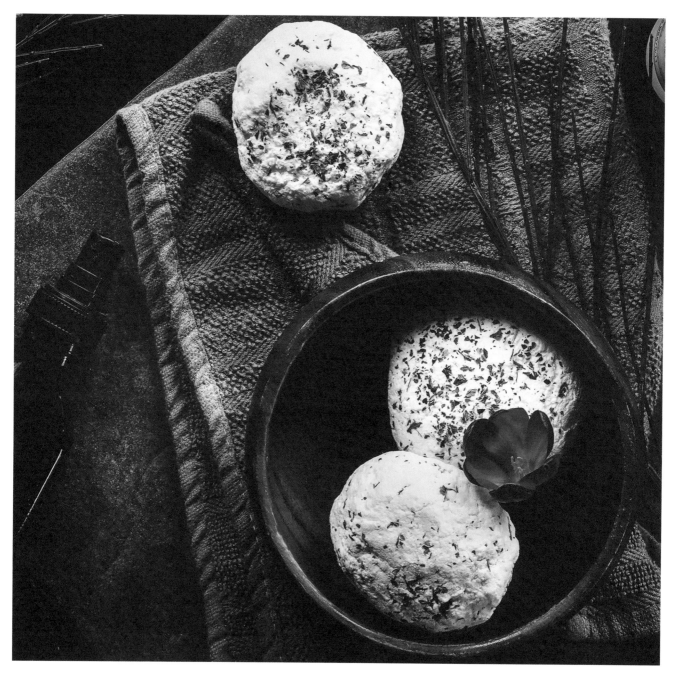

Bring the benefits of aromatherapy to bath time even when you don't have a tub.

SHOWER BOMB
with MENTHOL

Makes 4 medium bombs

Using strong menthol crystals in bath products is not advisable. But shower bombs are wonderful vessels for aromatherapy and can contain sinus-opening ingredients that would be too strong for use in the bathtub.

DIRECTIONS

1. Add the baking soda and citric acid to a bowl and mix. Be sure to break up any clumps. Set aside.

2. Measure out the menthol crystals into double boiler over medium heat, and gently heat until the crystals have turned to liquid.

3. Remove from the heat and allow the menthol to cool slightly, then stir in the essential oils.

4. Slowly pour the melted mixture into the dry ingredients while stirring.

5. Use a fork to thoroughly incorporate and break up any clumps.

6. Fill a spray bottle with witch hazel and add by spraying it onto the baking soda mixture while stirring.

INGREDIENTS

1 cup baking soda

½ cup citric acid

3 Tablespoons organic menthol crystals

20 drops organic eucalyptus essential oil

10 drops organic rosemary essential oil

⅛ cup organic witch hazel extract

Organic peppermint, spearmint, or eucalyptus leaf (optional decorations)

Continued ➜

7. Once the mixture holds together on its own, scoop out one-quarter of the mixture and pat it into a sphere. Pack it well so that the bomb will not crumble as it dries.

8. Sprinkle some of the optional decorations on the top and gently push in so the herbs stick.

9. Place on parchment paper to dry for 24 hours.

10. Store the shower bombs in containers in a cool, dry space.

TO USE

1. Heat up the shower water.

2. Once you are ready to get in, add the shower bomb. We like to keep the bomb slightly outside of the water to extend its aromatherapeutic qualities.

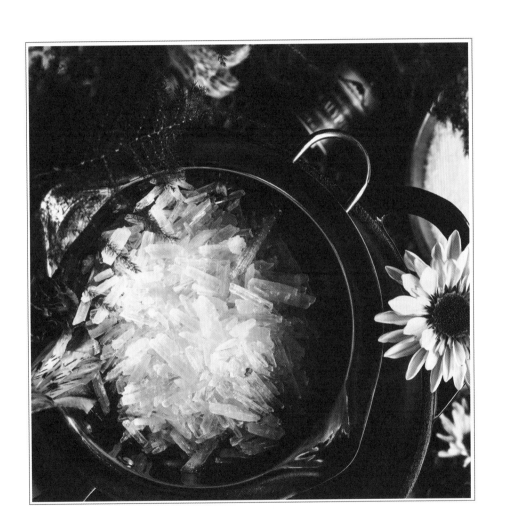

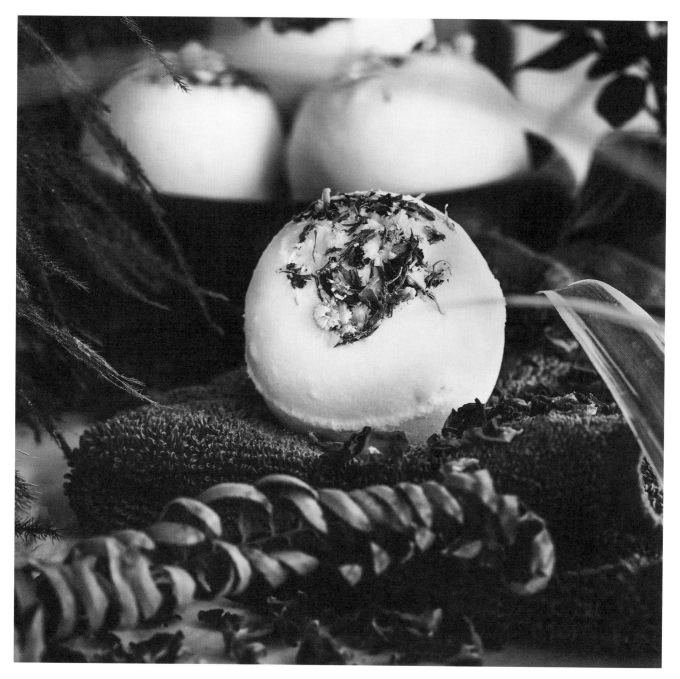

Bath bombs offer aromatic bliss whenever you need to leave the world outside the door.

FLORAL BATH BOMBS

Makes 4 medium bombs

The finicky part of making bath bombs is getting the moisture level right—the bombs should be able to sit up on their own while they are still wet. Make these floral bath bombs ahead of time, so when you need to relax you can sink right in.

DIRECTIONS

1. Thoroughly mix the baking soda and citric acid together in a bowl, being sure to break up the clumps.

2. Add optional flowers of choice until fully blended. Set aside.

3. In a separate small bowl, whisk together the sunflower oil and essential oils.

4. While stirring constantly, slowly pour the oil mixture into the dry ingredients.

5. Once incorporated, slowly mist the mixture with witch hazel while stirring. Be sure not to oversaturate the mixture with witch hazel: when you're able to clump the mixture in your hands without it falling apart, it is ready to shape.

6. You can use bath bomb molds, measuring cups, or even your hands to form the bombs.

7. Place the bath bombs on parchment paper to dry for 2 days.

8. Put the dried bombs into clean, dry storage containers, and store in a cool, dry place until ready to use.

INGREDIENTS

2 cups baking soda

1 cup citric acid

1 heaping Tablespoon organic rose petals, dried or fresh (optional)

1 heaping Tablespoon organic cornflowers or lavender flowers, dried or fresh (optional)

2 Tablespoons organic sunflower oil

10 drops organic lavender essential oil

5 drops organic ylang ylang essential oil

Organic witch hazel extract in a spray bottle for misting

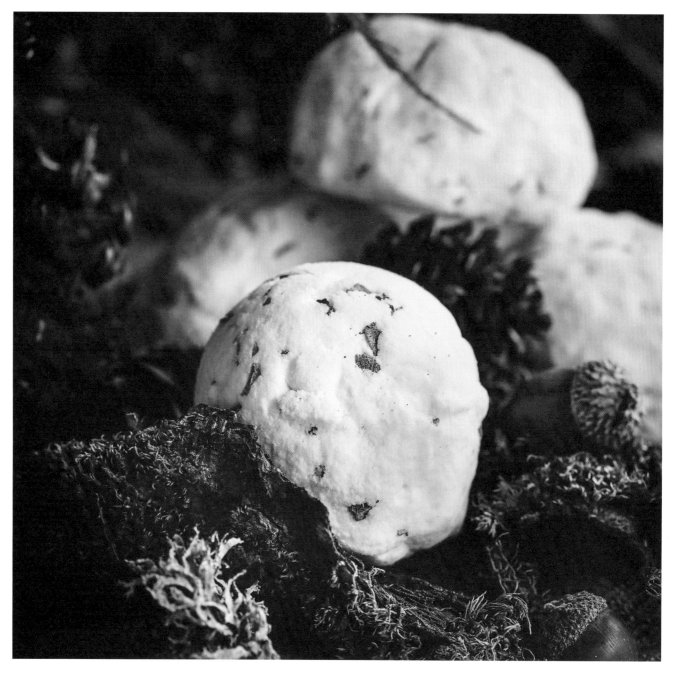

Bring the principles of energetic forest bathing to your bath.

WOODLAND ESCAPE BATH BOMBS

Makes 4 medium bombs

Because bath bombs are crafted in advance, they are an easy way to enjoy aromatherapy after a long day. Hand-forming bath bombs creates a rougher surface, which goes well with the rustic woodland theme of this recipe.

INGREDIENTS

2 cups baking soda

1 cup citric acid

2 heaping Tablespoons organic culinary sage leaves (optional)

2 Tablespoons organic sunflower oil

10 drops Virginia cedarwood essential oil

4 drops organic black spruce essential oil

3 drops organic sage essential oil

Organic witch hazel extract in a spray bottle for misting

DIRECTIONS

1. Thoroughly mix the baking soda and citric acid in a bowl, making sure to break up clumps.

2. Add the sage leaves and stir to fully incorporate. Set aside.

3. In a separate small bowl, whisk together the sunflower oil and essential oils.

4. While stirring constantly, slowly pour the oil mixture into the dry ingredients.

5. Once incorporated, slowly mist the mixture with witch hazel as you stir. Be sure not to oversaturate the mixture with witch hazel: when you're able to clump the mixture in your hands without it falling apart, it is ready to shape.

6. You can use bath bomb molds, measuring cups, or your hands to form the bombs.

7. Place the bath bombs on parchment paper to dry for 2 days.

8. Put the dried bombs into clean, dry storage containers, and store in a cool, dry place until ready to use.

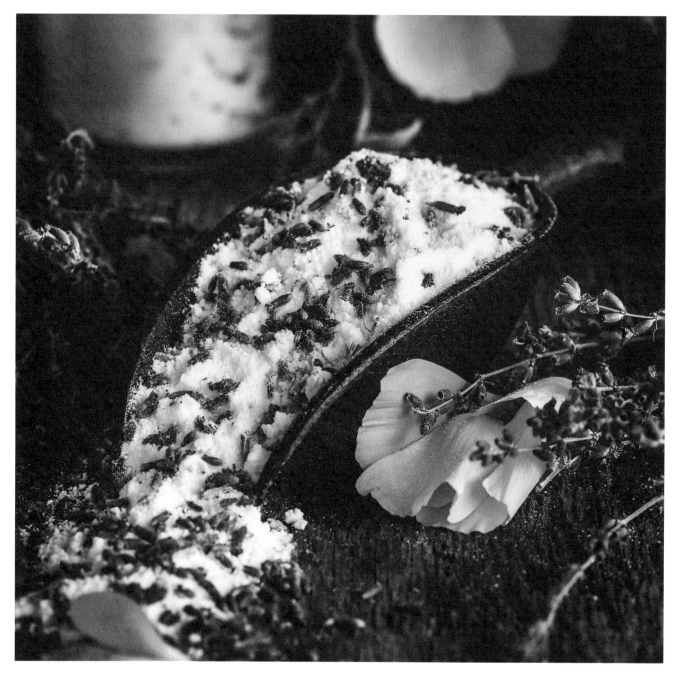

A fizzing bath mix offers a quick path to relaxation.

FIZZY BATH MIX

Makes enough for 1 bath

This fizzy bath mix gives you all the fun and soothing qualities of a bath bomb, without having to make the bombs or wait for them to dry.

INGREDIENTS

¾ cup baking soda

20 drops organic lavender essential oil

¼ cup citric acid

1 Tablespoon organic lavender flowers (optional)

1 teaspoon organic jojoba oil

DIRECTIONS

1. In a bowl, stir together the baking soda and lavender essential oil.

2. Add the citric acid, lavender flowers, and jojoba oil. Mix thoroughly.

TO USE

1. Fill the bathtub with warm water.

2. To take full advantage of the fizz, pour the mixture in the bath and get in immediately.

TIPS

This bath mix can be made ahead and stored for later use in an airtight container kept in a cool, dark, dry place.

This recipe can also be multiplied and stored in upcycled, decorative jars for gift giving.

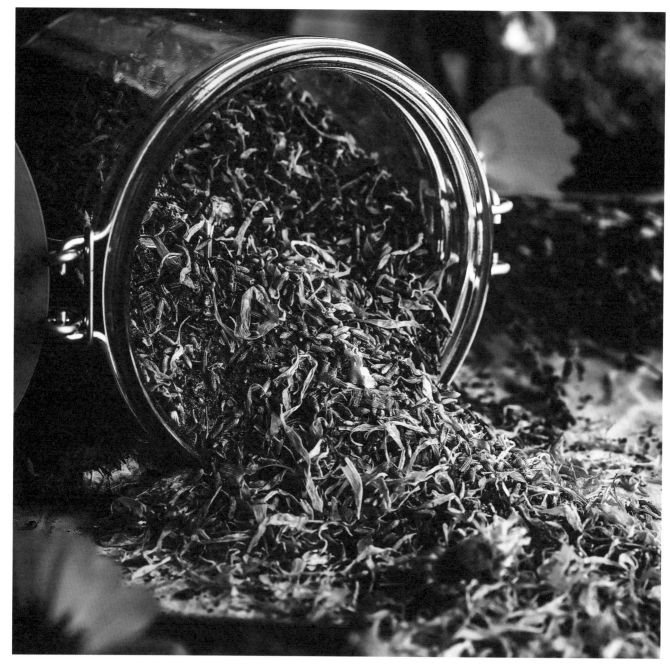

A classic herbal tea bath offers botanical support without having to prepare anything in advance.

HERBAL TEA BATH

You can take your bath experience to a new level by adding therapeutic herbs to customize your routine based on your specific needs and preferences. Keep a jar of herbs near the tub so you'll be ready to pamper yourself whenever the inspiration flows.

DIRECTIONS

1. Mix your choice of herbs in an airtight jar for storage.

2. When ready to use, fill a drawstring cotton muslin bag with the herbal blend and hang it on the faucet so hot water runs through the herbs and creates a tea in the tub.

3. Once the tub is full, toss the tied bag into the water and swish it around to infuse your bath with even more herbal goodness.

4. Alternatively, make a large pot of tea using your herbal bath blend and add that herbal infused liquid to the tub before getting in.

INGREDIENTS

Some of our favorite herbs for bathing include:

Calendula flowers

Chamomile flowers

Cleavers

Comfrey leaf

Ginger root

Holy basil leaf

Hops

Lavender flowers

Lemon balm leaf

Oat tops

Passionflower

Peppermint leaf

Red clover blossoms

Roses

Rosemary leaf

TIPS

Breaking or crushing large herbal flowers will create more botanical surface area and deliver more herbal goodness to your bath infusion.

If the herbs are already crushed or have fine particulates, it's normal for some herbs to get into the bath water.

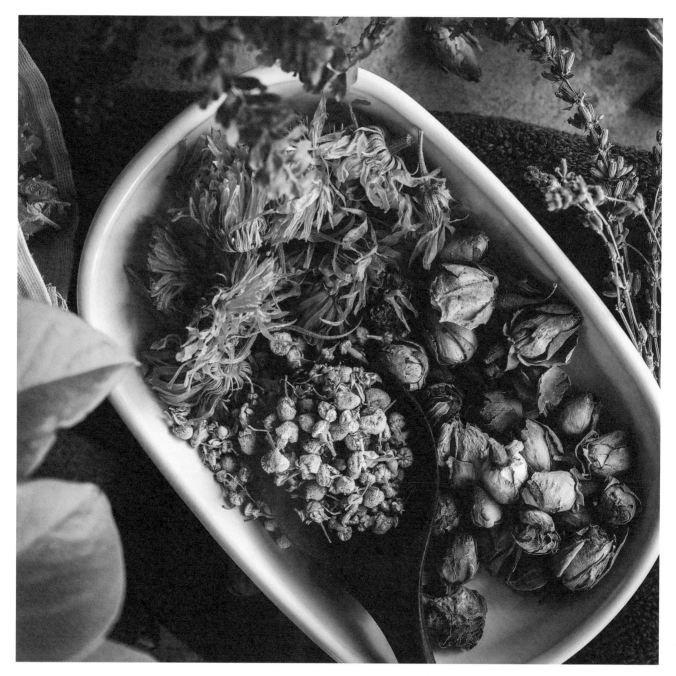

Calendula, chamomile, and rose are gentle enough for babies.

HERBAL BATH
FOR BABIES

Makes enough for 1 bath

Organic calendula and chamomile are gentle and nourish the skin. When combined with the soothing aromatics of lavender or roses, they make a perfect herbal bath for little ones and adults alike.

Organic chamomile flowers and/or calendula flowers

Organic lavender flowers, rose petals, or rose buds

DIRECTIONS

1. Play around with the proportion of herbs to see what works best for you. For beginners, start with equal parts chamomile and calendula and about half as much lavender or rose petals.

2. Fill a muslin bag, cotton tea net, or tea ball infuser with herbs of choice. Make sure to tie or seal the vessel well so the herbs don't spill into the bath water.

3. Put the bag or infuser directly into the bath water. Agitate and let the herbs infuse for 2 to 5 minutes before removing.

4. Your baby can relax in the herb-infused bath water for 10 to 20 minutes, fully supervised, so long as the water stays warm and comforting.

TIPS

One small muslin bag, cotton tea net, or tea ball is sufficient for a baby-size tub or the kitchen sink. For an adult bath, use a large muslin bag, tea ball infuser, or tea net, or double up on the small bag.

A muslin or cotton tea bag also makes a good washcloth for a baby's delicate skin.

Cue up some soothing music in the background and create an all-around relaxing sensory experience for bath time.

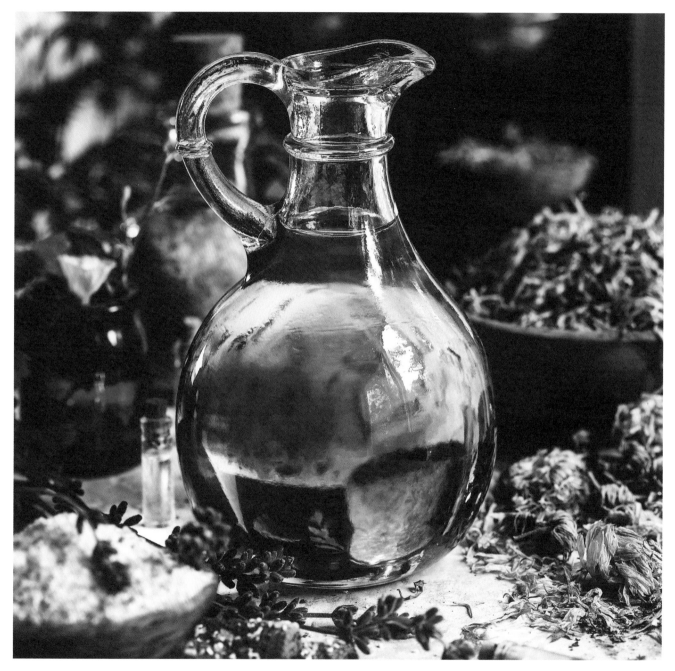

There's no better way to relax than in a warm bath with herb-infused oils.

AROMATIC BATH OIL

Makes about ½ cup

A warm bath with herb-infused oils helps to relax tense muscles, open pores, encourage digestion, soften the skin, and promote restful sleep. After a good soak, it's also lovely to spritz your skin and the air around you with cooling hydrosol.

INGREDIENTS

½ cup organic carrier oil

20 to 40 drops organic essential oil(s)

DIRECTIONS

1. Choose an organic carrier oil for your base. Jojoba, rosehip seed, kukui nut, or sweet almond oil are all good choices.

2. Select an essential oil that is safe for use in topical preparations and fitting for your particular mood or current need. If you want something relaxing, try lavender. If you want an uplifting scent, try sweet orange or geranium. Need to soothe the muscles? Try rosemary.

3. Put the carrier oil into a bottle that has a tight-fitting cap.

4. Slowly drip the essential oil(s) into the bottle, tighten the cap, and roll between your palms to blend.

5. Store the oil in a cool dark place between uses.

TO USE

1. Add 1 to 2 teaspoons of the oil blend to a filled tub and swirl throughout the water before getting in.

2. Keep the oil well dispersed as you bathe.

3. Be careful when exiting the tub, because oil-based bath recipes can create a slipping hazard.

TIPS

For a sweet addition, infuse the carrier oil base with an organic vanilla bean for 2 weeks before blending with the essential oils.

1 teaspoon of organic unrefined coconut oil melted into your bath water is also an easy and lovely option!

8

Herbal Remedies for Common Ailments

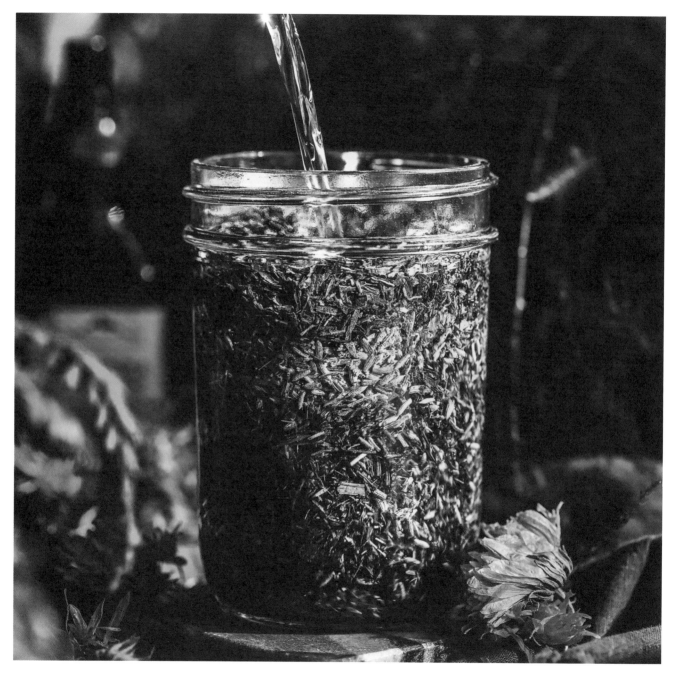

The skin-loving properties of green tea harmonize with soothing aloe vera and calendula to provide after-sun comfort.

NATURAL AFTER-SUN SPRAY *with* CALENDULA

Makes about ¾ cup

This after-sun spray combines the generous cooling benefits of aloe vera with infused witch hazel extract and skin-loving calendula hydrosol to cool and refresh the skin after spending time in the sun.

STEP ONE DIRECTIONS

1. Fill half a 7-ounce or larger pantry jar with a mixture of equal parts green tea leaves, lavender, and cleavers. (You'll need at least a ½ cup of finished extract for this recipe, but feel free to make more and save it for other projects.)

2. Pour the witch hazel extract over the herbs to fill the jar.

3. Put on an airtight lid, shake well, and allow to infuse for 2 to 4 weeks.

4. Strain into a pantry jar and label with the name and date for future use.

5. Store in the refrigerator. Infused witch hazel should last several months.

Step 1: Make Infused Witch Hazel Extract

Organic dried green tea leaves

Organic dried lavender flowers

Organic dried cleavers

Organic witch hazel extract

Step 2: Make After-Sun Spray

½ cup homemade infused witch hazel extract

¼ cup organic calendula hydrosol (cucumber, rose, or peppermint hydrosols are other good options)

⅛ cup organic aloe vera gel

Continued →

STEP TWO DIRECTIONS

1. In a glass bottle with a mister, combine the herb-infused witch hazel extract with the hydrosol and aloe vera gel.

2. Secure the mister cap, shake well, and spray generously on your skin as needed. Avoid contact with your eyes and other sensitive areas.

3. Keep refrigerated. This spray will last up to a year if properly stored.

TIPS

This spray may help deal with occasions of over-sunning, but it is not an excuse to forget about sun safety! We encourage everyone to take appropriate UV precautions whenever possible, such as limiting periods of direct exposure and wearing protective coverings.

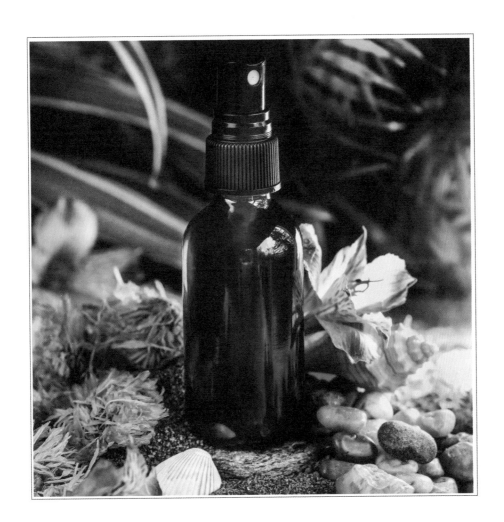

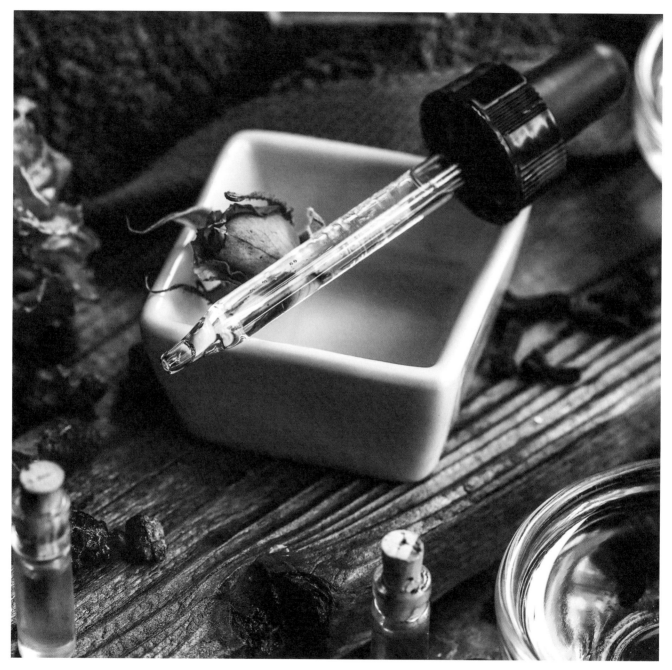

Fungus-fighting nail oil is easy to apply and quickly absorbs into the affected areas.

FUNGUS-FIGHTING ROSE NAIL OIL

Makes about ½ cup

This nail oil brings the powers of roses, tea tree, and clove bud to the battle against nail fungus and simultaneously delivers vitamins and essential fatty acids to strengthen and moisturize your nails and cuticles.

DIRECTIONS

1. Combine the argan and jojoba oils with the rose petals and infuse using either the solar or quick heat method.

2. Strain the rose petals from the oil mixture and allow it to cool.

3. Combine the rose-infused oil with tea tree oil, clove bud or myrrh oil, and vitamin E oil in a storage bottle with an airtight lid. Seal well and agitate the bottle to fully combine.

4. Put a portion of the nail oil in a smaller bottle with a dropper lid for use.

5. Store both bottles in a cool, dark place.

INGREDIENTS

2 Tablespoons organic argan oil

2 Tablespoons organic jojoba oil

¼ cup organic rose petals

24 drops organic tea tree essential oil

6 drops organic clove bud essential oil or 12 drops organic myrrh essential oil

5 drops vitamin E oil

TIPS

This is a process that requires consistency and patience. In the meantime, your nails and cuticles will love the attention.

Continued ➜

1. Wash your hands or feet, including the nails, with soap and warm water. You can use a soft toothbrush to thoroughly scrub around your toes and cuticles. Dry thoroughly.

2. Shake the dropper bottle to recombine the oils. Apply a few drops of the nail oil blend to the affected nail(s).

3. Let the oil soak in, which this may take several minutes.

4. Repeat daily. If you are not experiencing discomfort or irritation from the oil, you can repeat morning and night. If you are experiencing discomfort, discontinue use.

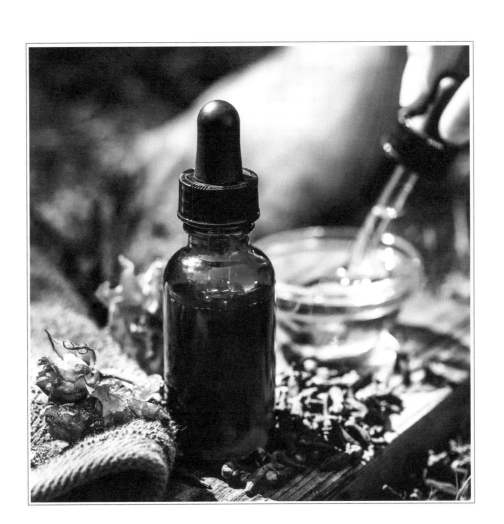

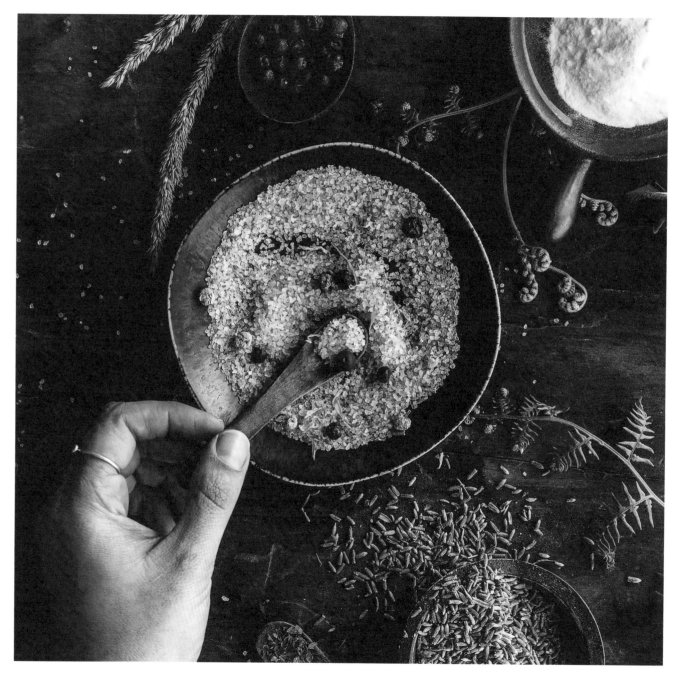

A sitz bath is ideal for easing general lower-body soreness and fatigue.

HERBAL SITZ BATH

Makes enough for 1 bath

A sitz bath is a shallow bath in which you can add salts, herbs, and other ingredients to create a clean, warm, healing pool in which to soak. There are small tubs made specifically for this purpose, which are ideal for concentrating the salts and herbs where you need them most. However, when dealing with pain and fatigue that impact the lower back and legs, a bathtub is the appropriate vessel.

Herbs for a sitz bath may be used dried, powdered, or chopped fresh. Some of our favorites include:

- › Arnica flowers
- › Calendula flowers
- › Chamomile flowers
- › Comfrey leaf
- › Eucalyptus leaf
- › Ginger root
- › Juniper berries
- › Lavender flowers
- › Mint leaf
- › Mustard seed
- › Rosemary leaf
- › Sage leaf
- › St. John's wort leaf

DIRECTIONS

1. Thoroughly scrub your bathtub and rinse it well so there is no soap residue.

2. Adjust water temperature so that it is warm enough to dissolve the salt but is not uncomfortably hot.

INGREDIENTS

1 to 2 cups Epsom salt per gallon of water, depending on skin sensitivity

½ to ¾ cup baking soda per gallon of water

Up to 1 cup other salts like Himalayan pink salt (optional)

Cotton tea net or muslin bag full of organic herbs of choice (approximately ½ cup)

TIPS

If you need to fill the tub a little deeper to reach your lower back, adjust the amount of Epsom salt, baking soda, and herbs accordingly for more water.

You can put herbs directly into your bath water, but cleaning them out again can be a pain in your just-soaked backside. A tea net or muslin bag makes cleanup a breeze. If you are using powdered herbs, you'll need to use a muslin bag.

Continued ➜

3. Fill the tub with just enough warm water so it will cover your hips when you sit down. Do not add other oils or soaps.

4. Add Epsom salt, baking soda, optional additional salts, and the bag of herbs. Agitate as necessary to dissolve the salts and baking soda and to encourage herbal goodness to seep into the bath. Alternatively, hang the herb bag on the spout so the water runs over it as the tub fills.

5. Climb in and soak for 15 to 20 minutes, making sure to keep the most affected areas of your lower body in the water.

6. Rinse off with fresh water. Gently pat yourself dry.

7. Repeat up to 3 to 4 times a day, as needed for relief.

Remember to rinse the tub after your sitz bath so you don't leave salt behind for the next person.

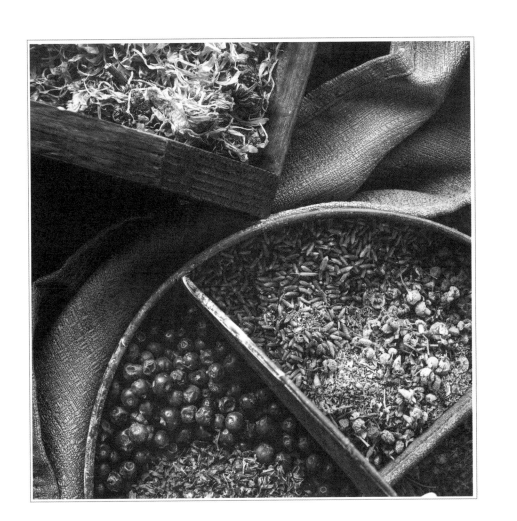

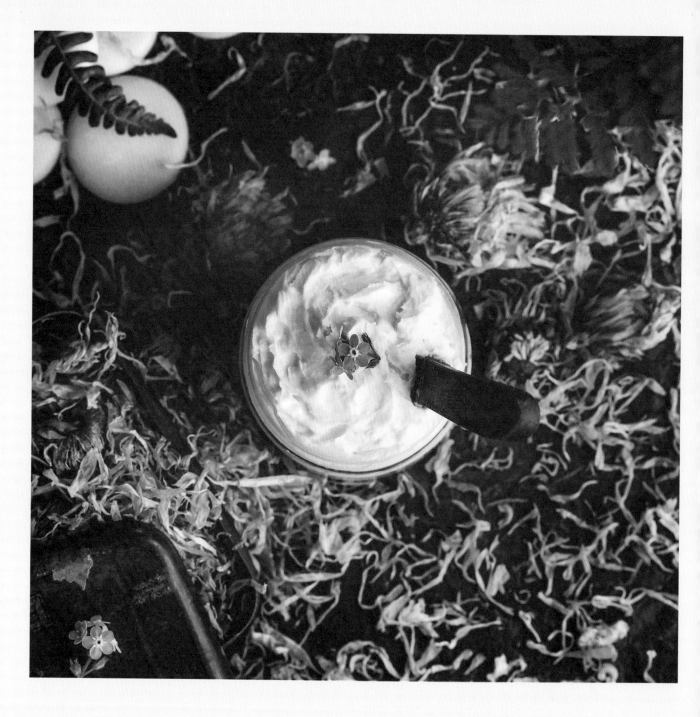

HERBAL SALVES

Herbal salves are a simple, effective, and enjoyable way to bring herbal goodness to your skin care regime. One of our favorite things about salves is that they are semi-solid at room temperature but soften when applied to the skin. This means they can be used for a wide variety of topical uses, are handy to store in tins, and can be kept in a purse or pocket without creating a mess—offering a handy way to protect, soothe, or nourish your skin wherever and whenever you want. Salves also make great gifts.

Step 1: Make Herb-Infused Oil

You can make a salve with a single herb or multiple herbs, depending on your project. It's useful to make a variety of herb-infused oils and keep them at the ready so you can easily craft a salve whenever you need it!

If you intend to use this infused oil only for topical use, you can infuse it by using any of the three oil infusion methods. However, if you also want to utilize the oil for culinary use, use either the solar or quick heat method.

TIPS

Using dried herbs rather than fresh will make infused oils more shelf stable.

If you are excited to begin making salves but don't have the time or inclination to infuse oil, feel free to purchase premade herb-infused oils.

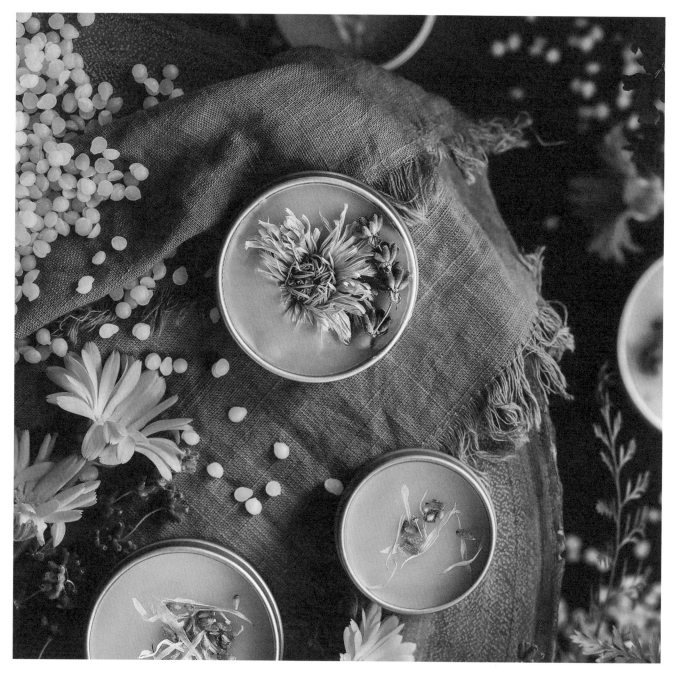

This calendula salve has wonderful skin-softening properties.

CALENDULA SALVE
with BEESWAX

Makes about ½ cup

This calendula salve is an exceptional blend for restoring working hands and for rubbing on tired muscles after a long workday. It also makes a good lip balm for chapped lips and is equally helpful for other minor skin irritations—because calendula is amazing like that!

INGREDIENTS

2 Tablespoons beeswax pastilles or grated beeswax

½ cup organic calendula-infused oil

10 to 20 drops lavender essential oil or other essential oil(s) of choice (optional)

3 to 4 drops vitamin E oil (optional)

DIRECTIONS

1. Gently heat the beeswax and oil in a double boiler over medium heat, swirling or stirring occasionally to blend, until the beeswax melts.

2. Remove from the heat and add the optional essential oil(s) and vitamin E oil.

3. Quickly pour the warm mixture into prepared tins, glass jars, or lip balm tubes and allow to cool completely.

4. Store in a cool location for 1 to 3 years.

TIPS

The consistency of salves can be adjusted by using less beeswax for a softer salve and more beeswax for a firmer salve. Consistency Test: Place a couple of clean metal spoons in the freezer before you begin. When the beeswax is melted, dip one of the frozen spoons into the pot and place it back into the freezer for 1 to 2 minutes. This will simulate the final consistency, and you can then adjust to suit your preferences.

To scale this recipe up or down, simply use 1 part beeswax to 4 parts of herb-infused oil.

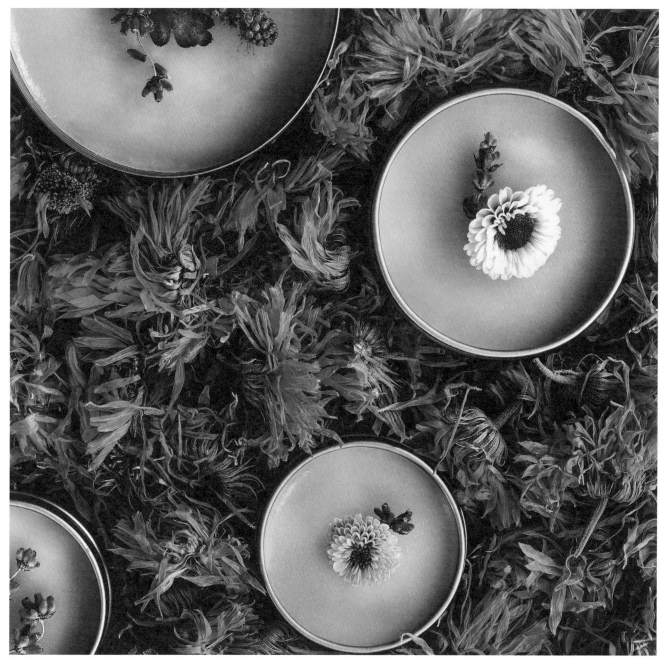

*Vegan salve, made with carnauba wax and luxurious butters, is
perfect for hydrating and softening dry, rough skin.*

VEGAN SALVE *with* CARNAUBA WAX

Makes about ½ cup

Carnauba wax is one of the hardest natural waxes available. It creates a salve that is extremely durable with a lovely glossy finish. Carnauba wax can be somewhat brittle when used by itself, but it softens nicely when combined with natural butters and is a particularly good choice if you prefer your salves to be on the firmer side. Due to its hardness, carnauba wax is not a one-to-one swap with beeswax in formulations. When substituting, it is also important to keep in mind that carnauba wax is typically combined with plant-based butters.

INGREDIENTS

3 Tablespoons organic calendula-infused oil

2 Tablespoons organic mango butter

1 Tablespoon kokum butter

1 Tablespoon + 1 teaspoon organic carnauba wax

¼ teaspoon vitamin E oil

9 drops organic lavender essential oil

9 drops organic Roman chamomile essential oil

DIRECTIONS

1. Place the calendula oil, butters, and wax in a double boiler over medium heat, and slowly and gently melt the butters and wax.

2. Once the ingredients are fully melted, remove from the heat and quickly stir in the vitamin E oil and essential oils.

3. Immediately pour the mixture into jars or tins, as it will start to set as soon as you remove it from the heat.

4. Allow the salve to fully set at room temperature before putting on the lids or using it. Because carnauba is a slow-setting wax, we like to give this salve 3 days to set.

5. When stored in a cool, dark place, this salve will last up to 2 years.

TIPS

Carnauba wax has a melting point of about 180°F, which means it can take a while for it to melt.

Rushing this process may scald the oils, so be sure to heat the mixture slowly.

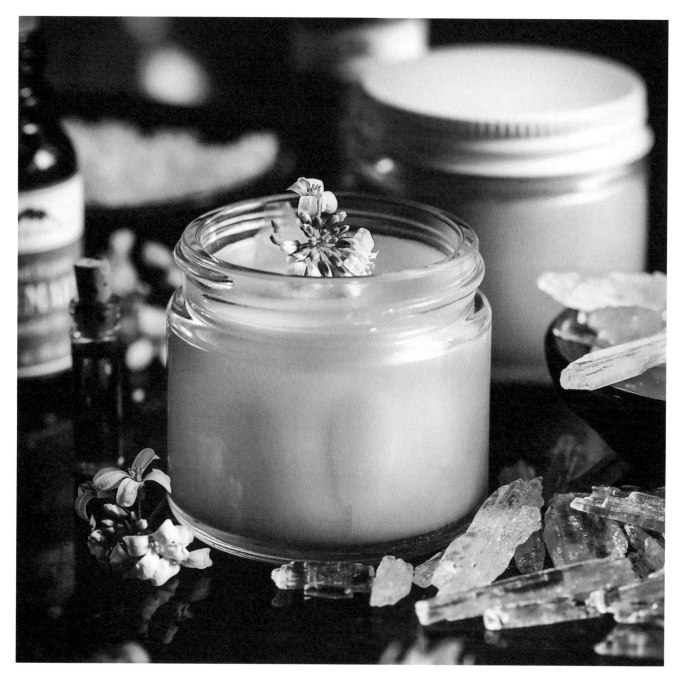

A mentholated chest rub is a staple preparation for your home wellness kit.

MENTHOL VAPOR CHEST RUB

Makes about 1 ⅛ cups

Eucalyptus, menthol, and rosemary come together in this mentholated rub to offer the perfect cooling, soothing trifecta.

Continued →

DIRECTIONS

1. Measure the carrier oil into the top of a double boiler.

2. For a more solid balm texture, use ⅛ cup of beeswax. If you prefer a texture closer to an ointment, use less.

3. Gently heat the oil and beeswax in the double boiler over medium heat until the beeswax melts.

4. When melted, remove from the heat and stir in the menthol crystals and essential oils until dissolved. For a stronger formulation, use the full 1 teaspoon of crystals. For a gentler one, use half.

5. Promptly pour into jars or tins.

6. Allow the mixture to completely cool before putting on the lids.

INGREDIENTS

1 cup organic carrier oil (medium absorption oils like olive, almond, coconut, or babassu are good choices)

⅛ cup beeswax pastilles or grated beeswax

½ to 1 teaspoon organic menthol crystals

20 drops organic eucalyptus essential oil

10 drops organic rosemary essential oil

TIPS

Store menthol crystals safely away from children and animals.

Always work in a well-ventilated area when using menthol crystals, or wear a mask if you find inhaling the aroma irritating.

This recipe errs on the safe side with a 2 percent content of menthol crystals. Menthol crystals can make up to 5 percent

TO USE

1. Rub a layer of balm on your chest and throat.

2. Cover with a warm, dry cloth if you'd like. As well as being comforting, the cloth protects clothing and sheets.

3. Wear something loose to allow the vapors to reach your nose.

4. Relax and breathe.

of a finished product for topical use, so you could add up to 2 teaspoons of the crystals. But keep in mind that they are strong.

Consult with your child's doctor before using a menthol or chest rub on children.

Menthol eucalyptus rub is for external use only. Do not put in eyes, mouth, nostrils, under bandages, or on damaged skin.

We always recommend applying a small patch test on your skin before using any product you have not used before.

Do not heat or microwave the chest rub before use.

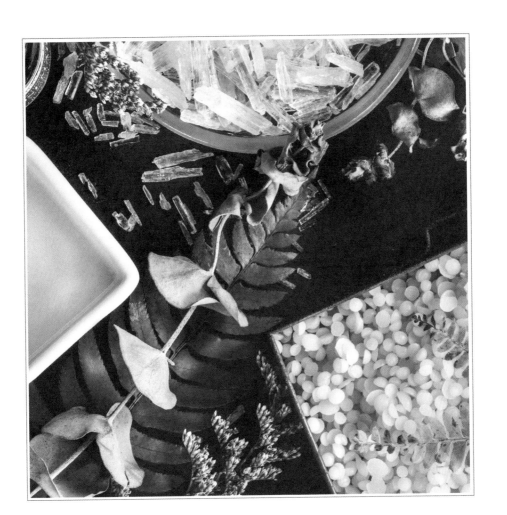

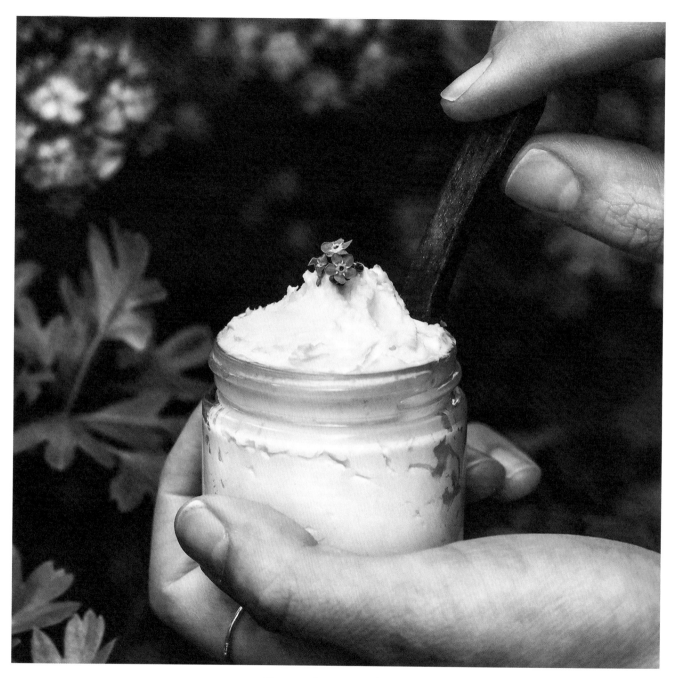

This cream brings serious botanical support to nipples that are working hard to feed a child.

SORE NIPPLES NURSING SALVE

Makes about ½ cup

Fractionated coconut oil is lightweight and fast absorbing, which makes it ideal for a nipple cream. You want to avoid using heavier oils or butters that leave your skin slick because it can affect how well your baby can latch on. Sunflower oil is a good substitute if you don't have fractionated coconut oil. Additionally, we opt not to use any form of wax in a nipple cream because it can leave a residue on the skin that goes into the child's mouth.

INGREDIENTS

2 Tablespoons organic refined shea butter

10 wafers organic roasted cocoa butter

2 Tablespoons organic calendula herbal oil

2 Tablespoons organic fractionated coconut oil

½ teaspoon vitamin E oil

DIRECTIONS

1. Combine the shea butter, cocoa butter, calendula oil, and fractionated coconut oil in the top of a double boiler over medium heat. Gently heat and stir until the butters liquify.

2. Remove from the heat and stir in the vitamin E oil.

3. Pour the mixture into a bowl and put it in the refrigerator.

4. When the mixture is starting to solidify near the center (the edges will solidify first), whip with a hand mixer to stiff peaks. If the mixture is not coming together, it can help to put the bowl in an ice bath and then whip.

TIPS

If you try to whip the mixture and it's still too liquid, put it back in the refrigerator. Keep an eye on it at that point because it often sets up quickly.

Continued →

1. Let your nipples air dry or pat them dry after nursing.

2. Rub a small dollop of nipple cream between your fingers—it doesn't take very much because this spreads nicely with body heat—and gently smooth onto your nipples and areolas.

3. If you are concerned about getting cream on your clothing, put a nursing pad or cloth inside your bra.

4. If the cream has not soaked into your skin when your baby wants to nurse next, know that the ingredients are edible and safe. However, if you have any concerns or if there is still residue, feel free to wipe it away to make sure your baby can latch on well.

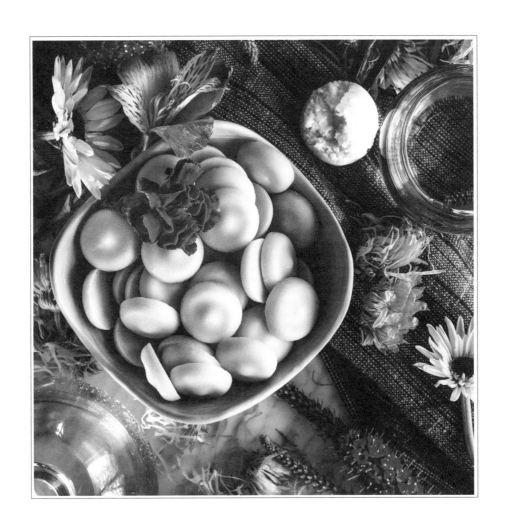

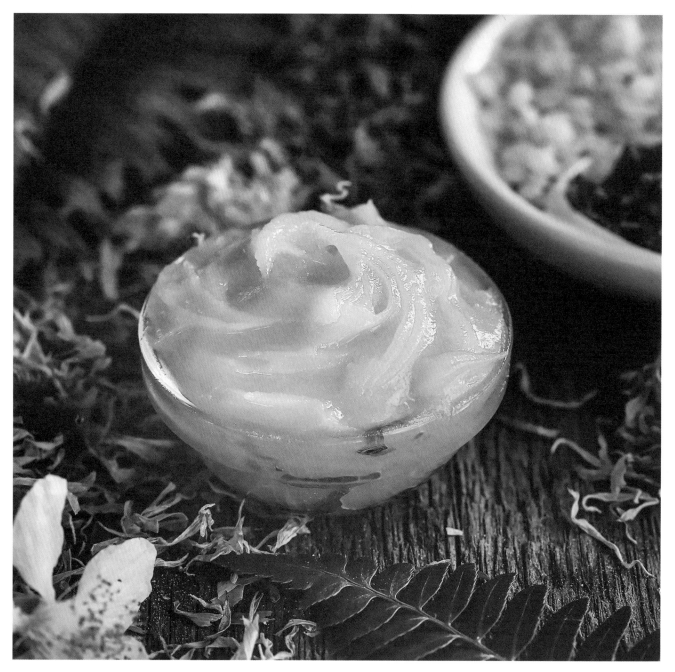

A simple diaper ointment made with olive oil, calendula, Oregon grape root, beeswax, and vitamin E can make all the difference when it comes to baby's comfort.

HERBAL DIAPER RASH OINTMENT

Makes about 1 cup

Calendula and Oregon grape root have proven themselves to be gentle and effective at protecting and soothing not just babies' diapered bottoms, but also adult skin irritations and minor scrapes.

INGREDIENTS

½ cup organic calendula-infused olive oil

½ cup organic Oregon grape–infused olive oil

¼ cup beeswax pastilles or grated beeswax

6 drops vitamin E oil (optional)

DIRECTIONS

1. In the top of a double boiler over medium heat, combine the oils and beeswax. Gently heat until the beeswax melts and the mixture is incorporated.

2. Remove from the heat and stir in the optional vitamin E oil.

3. Pour into tins or glass jars. Allow the salve to cool completely before placing lids on the containers.

4. Store in a cool, dry place. If stored properly, salves can last 2 to 3 years.

Index

MOUNTAIN ROSE HERBS

Founded in 1987 by the "godmother of herbalism," Rosemary Gladstar, Mountain Rose Herbs has grown from a small mail-order business into a company that is renowned as one of the largest organic bulk herbs distributors in the nation. As well as being a primary source of ethically grown and harvested organic herbs, spices, teas, essential oils, and botanical goods, Mountain Rose Herbs is a go-to source for herbal education and they have spent more than three decades inspiring thousands of herbalists, educators, and DIY body care crafters.

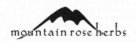